Fresh Fruit CLEANSE

Fresh Fruit CLEANSE

Detox, Lose Weight and Restore Your Health with Nature's Most Delicious Foods

Leanne Hall

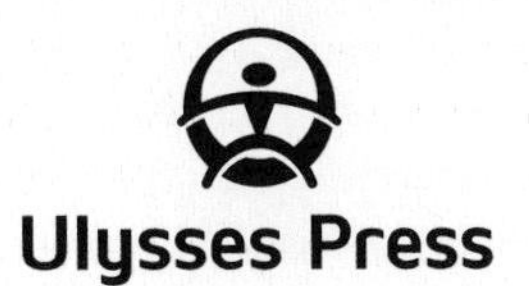

Ulysses Press

Published in the U.S. by
ULYSSES PRESS
P.O. Box 3440
Berkeley, CA 94703
www.ulyssespress.com

ISBN13: 978-1-56975-922-6
Library of Congress Control Number 2011922518

Acquisitions Editor: Keith Riegert
Managing Editor: Claire Chun
Editor: Susan Lang
Copyeditor: Elyce Petker
Proofreaders: Lauren Harrison, Abigail Reser
Production: Judith Metzener
Front cover design: what!design @ whatweb.com
Cover photos: © Dudarev Mikhail / shutterstock.com

Printed in the United States by Bang Printing

10 9 8 7 6 5 4 3 2 1

Distributed by Publishers Group West

NOTE TO READERS
This book has been written and published strictly for informational and educational purposes only. It is not intended to serve as medical advice or to be any form of medical treatment. You should always consult your physician before altering or changing any aspect of your medical treatment and / or undertaking a diet regimen, including the guidelines as described in this book. Do not stop or change any prescription medications without the guidance and advice of your physician. Any use of the information in this book is made on the reader's good judgment after consulting with his or her physician and is the reader's sole responsibility. This book is not intended to diagnose or treat any medical condition and is not a substitute for a physician.

Contents

Acknowledgments 7

Foreword 10

Part I: Getting Started

1 The Fresh Fruit Cleanse 15

2 Why Cleanse? 21

3 The Fresh Fruit Cleanse: Different from the Rest 31

Part II: Starting the Fresh Fruit Cleanse

4 Choosing the Best Fresh Fruit Cleanse for You 37

5 The Fresh Fruit Cleanse Menu 54

6 1-Day Fruit Blast 91

7 3-Day Reset Cleanse 93

8 5-Day Rebalance Cleanse 97

9 7-Day Detox Diet 103

10 The Nutritional Benefits of Fruit 111

11 Fruits by the Numbers 123

12 The Dirty Dozen and Buying Organic 151

Part III: Life after the Fresh Fruit Cleanse

13 After the Fresh Fruit Cleanse....159

14 Releasing Yourself from the Toxic Western Life....205

15 Life Practices: Changing the Little Things....217

16 Yoga....224

17 Inspirations and Affirmations to Live By....233

18 Conclusion....237

Appendix

Testimonials....240

References....244

About the Author....248

Acknowledgments

Thank you to my parents for their awesome love and belief in me. To my father for igniting his passion for love, life, and all things good into me, and for cheering me on all along the way. To my mother for the grace, wisdom, and faith she has shined on my life, for seeing the light in me and leading me to my faith in God's love with her everpresent unconditional love and support. Thank you to my family for loving me so graciously and being there for me. Thank you to all my teachers who have shined their light into my life. From Jesus Christ to Paramahansa Yogananda, and many beloved guides throughout my life, including Reverend David Norling, Reverend David Roseberry, and the incredible friends who have blessed my life from the time I was a child. And thank you to John Ponikvar for awakening in me a passion for writing; his joy and love of literature and the written word continue to inspire me. I am grateful for the spiritual community of love and friendship that lifts me up to heal and be strengthened with God's grace and love each day. And I am so grateful to Ulysses Press for believing in me and giving me this chance to share my story. It is one of healing and passion for health and well-being, and I hope it touches the lives of others in a positive way. For all of you who have blessed my life with your guidance, friendship, and love, I am eternally grateful. Thank you.

The Fruit Tree Planting Foundation

To celebrate the release of *Fresh Fruit Cleanse,* Ulysses Press will make a donation to the Fruit Tree Planting Foundation, a nonprofit charity dedicated to planting edible, fruitful trees and plants to benefit the environment and all its inhabitants. Their primary mission is to plant a collective total of 18 billion fruit trees across the world—approximately three for every person alive—and encourage their growth under organic standards.

Fruit trees heal the environment by cleaning the air, improving soil quality, preventing erosion, creating animal habitats, sustaining valuable water sources and providing healthy nutrition. The foundation's programs are at the forefront of a global sustainability movement by strategically donating orchards where the harvest will best serve communities for generations. Such places are: public schools, city parks, low-income neighborhoods, Native American reservations, international hunger relief sites and animal sanctuaries.

> May mankind instead of hunting for gold, racing for fame, or wasting productive forces in useless labors: choose the better part: the peaceful emulation in the discovery and direction of the natural forces for evolving nutritive products and the peaceable enjoyment of the fruits which the earth is able to produce in abundance for all.
>
> May man use his divine heritage of reason to attain true happiness by discovering the sources whence all earthly blessings flow and thus put an end to self-seeking and greed, to the increasing difficulties of making a living, the anxieties for the daily bread, to distress and crime—such is the aim of this little work, and in this may God aid us!
>
> —*Julius Hensel,* Bread from Stones, *October 1, 1893*

Thank you for your contribution to this positive cause and for helping to make the world a better and healthier place. To learn more about the Fruit Tree Planting Foundation or to make a donation to this wonderful cause, please visit www.ftpf.org.

Foreword

When I was asked to write *Fresh Fruit Cleanse,* I was still recovering from the difficult loss of my father just a year and half earlier. I was growing stronger but still healing emotionally and physically. Although I had been through several fruit cleanses over the previous nine years, I experienced significant healing by developing and going through the Fresh Fruit Cleanse while writing this book. The incredible recipes I discovered helped me to find the much-needed healing and nourishment I had been seeking. I feel so much stronger and healthier now. Before starting on this book, I didn't fully realize just how powerful the God-given medicinal power of food could be.

I've been on the path of wellness since taking my first yoga class in 2001. In 2003, I attended a weeklong seminar featuring some of the greatest health and wellness experts in the world, and I gained information that transformed me. I learned about "super foods" and began to wonder about the medicinal power of food. But at that time I didn't fully or consistently integrate those foods into my lifestyle. I dabbled in super foods, but more often than not, the unhealthier choices I was making in my life won over and I gave into them.

I had been through some difficult times before losing my father, but his death was the most difficult of all. I knew I must commit to change if I wanted a healthier, better life. When the offer came to write this book, I was thrilled, yet I didn't realize how incredibly therapeutic working on the book would be. Gandhi said, "You must be the change you wish to see in the world." I wanted to be that change, but I wasn't being it fully. Challenges in life would arise, and I would give into my old habits and patterns. One step forward, two steps back. Now I realize there is no turning back. I realized that it is, in fact, more possible to enjoy pleasure in life when you are no longer controlled by the false idea that some pleasure, like food or alcohol, will give you lasting happiness—because no sensual pleasure is capable of providing any true lasting happiness or joy. That's why all of the spiritual teachings say we must know the light and love of God within ourselves through spiritually healing practices like yoga, cleansing, meditation, prayer, and the loving fellowship of family, friends, and spiritual community. True joy comes from sharing that light and love in service to others.

The Fresh Fruit Cleanse is so much more than a weight-loss and detox program with wonderful recipes. I hope you'll realize, as I did, that food has medicinal power. Food isn't something we are meant to overeat or something we're meant to go to the gym to burn off. Food is a miraculous and medicinal energy. Fruits, vegetables, whole grains, and super foods like spirulina, maca, and raw cacao are what we are meant to eat. We are meant to give our cells and bodies optimal nutrition if we want to be healthy and to feel great, look great, slow down the aging process, and reduce the risk of disease. When your cells feel juicy from healthy food, you will feel your best in body, mind, and spirit. *Let thy food be thy medicine and thy medicine be thy food.* Hippocrates said this in 400 BC, and it's just as true now as it was then. Truth doesn't change. It's timeless and eternal.

The journey of a thousand miles begins with a single step.
— *Lao Tzu*

Many of the steps I took over the years seemed small at first. My first fruit cleanse in 2002 was challenging, partly because I didn't have a thorough, supportive nutritional program like the one I created for this book. However, I continued to take steps forward, even though sometimes I fell back a couple of steps. My first yoga teacher would often remark that sometimes things have to get worse before they can get better. A step is still a step and it's about progress, not perfection. So, just keep stepping. Whatever positive changes you wish to make physically, mentally, emotionally, spiritually, and even professionally, you can do it. I know you can.

I'm so grateful I was able to write this book, because now there's a program that anyone can follow and successfully complete with ease. I hope you will benefit from the Fresh Fruit Cleanse and a healthy lifestyle. I'm so grateful to be able to share all of this with you.

May we all grow well and awaken to conscious health, vitality, and well-being. I wish you blessings of joy, peace, love, prosperity, and—most of all—health.

May the peace and love of God be with you.

PART I

Getting Started

1

The Fresh Fruit Cleanse

When our health improves, every other aspect of our life improves simultaneously.

—David Wolfe, nutritional expert and leading raw foodist

If you are reading this book, then you are inspired to make positive changes in your life. I hope the book will support you by giving you the guidance and tools you need to grow in the best and healthiest way possible and to awaken you to your true potential in body, mind, and spirit. We need the support of one another to grow well. One of my favorite sayings is, *environment is stronger than will.* This book will encourage you to eat well, live consciously, make better choices in your life, and discover a healthier environment and community so you are continuously strengthened and inspired to make the positive changes you desire for yourself. With healthy living practices, like the ones in this book, you can transform your health and live the life you love.

My Journey

I grew up in a beautiful small town called Chagrin Falls, outside Cleveland, Ohio. Although my parents lived a very healthy lifestyle and inspired me to be healthy, I still ate junk food as a kid. All the things you can imagine: pizza, soda (lots and lots of Mountain Dew), potato chips, sugar-filled cereals, you name it. I'm sure a lot of us ate like this as children or adolescents. As a child growing up in America, this diet is hard to avoid.

In my early teenage years, around the age of 13, I started to make some unhealthy choices my parents didn't know about. I began to drink alcohol and smoke cigarettes with my peers. While I was a good student who loved learning and cared about doing well in school, from then on, my friends and I spent a lot of time drinking and partying.

Live with Passion

If it weren't for my passions in life and the incredible parents who encouraged me, I'm not sure how I would have ever been inspired to become better physically, mentally, emotionally, spiritually, and professionally. So, even though I used unhealthy substances during my teenage and early adult years, my passions always helped me to stay on track, or get back on track, when I lost my focus.

I think what so many people are missing in life is a real sense of passion, or purpose, for living. Whenever I've found something that inspires me, I've always had a natural desire to grow and become the best I can be. I was passionate about gymnastics, ballet, cheerleading, horseback riding, and playing the piano during my childhood and teenage years. In college, I loved learning Spanish. Now my passion for yoga inspires me to stay on a healthy path.

Exercise

My alcohol use continued throughout college, and so did my unhealthy eating. I gained about 20 pounds—my heaviest—during my sophomore year, when I lived in Spain for three months. I didn't like how I felt or looked, so I decided to start exercising the following year. One of my roommates, a model who was really into exercise, nutrition, and healthy eating, inspired me. I wanted to look like her because she glowed and was beautiful. I started going to the gym regularly, but I really didn't like it at first. After a while I started to feel better and liked the changes I was seeing in my body. I began to consume healthier foods as well. I ate a really low-calorie, low-fat diet, and I lost the weight I had put on while living abroad. But I often felt as if I were starving myself, and I got bored eating the same foods, mostly salad, all the time. I was thin again, but I wasn't happy because I felt deprived.

> When you are inspired by some great purpose, some extraordinary project, all your thoughts break their bonds: Your mind transcends limitations, your consciousness expands in every direction, and you find yourself in a new, great, and wonderful world. Dormant forces, faculties and talents become alive, and you discover yourself to be a greater person by far than you ever dreamed yourself to be.
>
> —*Patanjali, founder of the system of yoga and author of* The Yoga Sutras of Patanjali

Yoga

After college, I was still working out regularly and staying in shape, but I was counting calories and struggling with my diet. I obsessively watched what I ate and was terrified of gaining weight. A couple of weeks before getting my first corporate job, I decided to try a yoga class. I had seen a magazine article about how a lot of celebrities were practicing yoga. I loved that first class. I felt completely toned, stretched, and cleansed, as if I had worked every muscle of my body. I started going to yoga class regularly. Soon my body was changing, too. My butt looked better than it ever had, my arms were getting toned, and my abs were gaining definition. I loved my body again, and I started feeling better, too. I noticed I could eat well without gaining weight.

After attending my yoga teacher's health workshop, I started to think differently about the foods I was eating. I realized I didn't like eating foods that made me feel heavy. I quit smoking cigarettes as well. As I began to feel healthier, I couldn't stand the taste and smell of cigarettes or the way smoking made me feel. I was able to quit drinking coffee, too. Again, I didn't like the way it made my body and mind feel—my skin was often irritated after drinking coffee, and I would feel jittery, too. I became more and more interested in yoga, healthy eating, and self-development. I realized I wasn't happy in my work, so after a lot of praying for guidance, I decided to leave my job in 2002 and teach yoga.

The Fresh Fruit Cleanse

Inspired by the changes in my life, I decided to do a fruit cleanse in 2002. It was really hard at first. Cleansing helps you to recognize and feel the emotions that linger beneath any addictive behaviors, such as overeating, consuming unhealthy foods, drinking excessively, smoking cigarettes, and drinking caffeine. I began to see that I was eating for emotional reasons. I would eat when I wasn't really hungry. I was suppressing frustration and feelings about experiences I had gone through in my life, and I was trying to get satisfaction or joy from food. But the more I tried to fill up with something outside myself, the emptier I felt. I began to realize that food, or material things, didn't make me feel happy, that happiness could only come from the inside. When I took compulsive eating out of my life by doing the cleanse, I began to realize how addicted I had been. Although it was difficult to see all of that at first, I am so glad I did.

I made it through my first fruit cleanse with five days of eating only avocados, tomatoes, and other fruits. Afterward, I felt better than I ever had before. That was only the beginning, though—lifestyle changes don't happen overnight. If you're like me, then you know the road to health and well-being can be a roller coaster ride. I went to wellness seminars and explored the world of motivational living and self-improvement, but at the same time I was making a lot of unhealthy choices. Yoga helped balance the unhealthy choices I made, but at times it was a struggle. I was still drinking quite a bit and eating unhealthy foods, even though I was also making some better choices for myself.

I realize now that a lot of my poor choices were influenced by the relationships I was in at the time. We definitely attract into our life the people we are being. As I mentioned, Gandhi said, "Be the change you wish to see in the world." The corollary to that is, be the person you wish to be in a relationship and that's whom you will attract. A minister and good friend of mine, Reverend Lee Wolak, says this: "Having a love relationship is never about finding someone who makes you feel good or completes you, it's about you feeling good and attracting those who are an energy match to you."

The road to wellness has been a journey, and it's one I'm grateful I've been able to take. Not only am I continuously inspired to grow well physically, mentally, and emotionally, but I'm also deeply inspired to grow well spiritually. As we heal from unhealthy habits and behaviors with healthy living practices like the Fresh Fruit Cleanse, yoga, exercise, and meditation, we can know the radiant health and blessings God intends for us. I hope the Fresh Fruit Cleanse and everything in this book will inspire you, too, to grow healthy and well in your body, mind, and spirit and to awaken you to your true potential with every breath you breathe.

> "For I know the plans I have for you," declares the Lord, "plans to prosper you and not to harm you, plans to give you hope and a future."
>
> —*Jeremiah 29:11*

Infinite blessings on your path to well-being.

2

Why Cleanse?

To lose one's health renders science null,
art inglorious, strength unavailing, wealth useless,
and eloquence powerless.
—Herophilus c. 300 BC

Good health is one of the greatest gifts there is. It is important to take the best care of your body that you can. Healthy practices like yoga, exercise, good nutrition, and the Fresh Fruit Cleanse will help you feel your very best not just in body but also in mind and spirit throughout your entire life.

Did you know there is a saying that disease begins on your plate? Even when you feel great, cleansing will still help you to detoxify and purify your body, mind, and heart. Over time, toxicity builds up in your cells no matter how healthy you are. Years of unhealthy eating and habits can damage your body's immune system and affect your energy and vitality. From time to time, it's essential to cleanse your body so you can renew, reenergize, and rebalance yourself on every level. The Fresh Fruit Cleanse will help you to do just that.

The Fresh Fruit Cleanse lasts anywhere from three to seven days, with a 1-Day Fruit Blast Cleanse recommended on a weekly or twice-monthly basis. Cleansing for longer periods than a day removes excess amounts of mucus from the intestinal walls and digestive tract, old fecal matter from the colon,

Benefits of the Fresh Fruit Cleanse

- Promotes healthy and safe weight loss
- Balances the nervous system
- Increases energy and revitalizes organs
- Cleanses and clears the skin for a glowing complexion
- Eases muscular and skeletal aches and pains for greater ease of movement, mobility, agility, flexibility, and strength
- Rejuvenates the digestive system
- Cleanses the colon and makes peristaltic action of the intestines stronger (the cause of a natural bowel movement)
- Detoxifies the body of fat cells, mucus, arterial cholesterol plaque, and those things that can cause disease, like worry and stress
- Restores metabolism and cell oxygenation
- Improves breathing, allowing you to breathe more efficiently and deeply
- Improves mental clarity and focus
- Redevelops a desire and taste for healthier foods
- Awakens confidence in the ability to control choices in life
- Reveals the body's innate healing and balancing potential
- Awakens real beauty on a cellular level on the inside and outside, allowing your inner light to shine

and trapped cellular waste, as well as inorganic mineral deposits that contribute to arthritis. Cleansing also purifies the liver, kidneys, and bloodstream. It enhances mental clarity, increases energy, and helps overcome addictions to food and substances like alcohol, coffee, and nicotine, as well as other unhealthy behaviors. Additionally, it reduces the stomach to its normal size, aiding in weight loss. A smaller stomach allows you to eat less and still feel full and satisfied from the healthy, nutritious food you are consuming. If you are able, allow yourself occasionally to cleanse for longer periods, up to ten days. Longer cleanses are even believed to help fight diseases, including chronic ones.

The better you care for your body, the better your quality of life will be, including relationships, work, joy, passions, activities, and everything else. If you want to make positive changes, the Fresh Fruit Cleanse is one of the most powerful ways to realign your body, mind, and spirit. Not only is cleansing a way to detoxify the body, but it's also an opportunity to reevaluate the choices you are making in life. Anytime you feel you are out of balance from eating unhealthy foods or making unhealthy choices, the Fresh Fruit Cleanse will help you to find a higher level of energy and vitality as well as better balance and well-being physically, mentally, emotionally, and spiritually. As you feel healthier you will be inspired to make better choices in all things, including what you eat, the people you spend time with, and the way you live this precious gift called life.

Before you begin your cleanse, ask yourself what changes you would like to make. Visualize yourself growing healthier and feeling inspired to be healthy and well. See yourself letting go of your unhealthy habits and growing into a healthier, happier person—and you will be amazed at what your positive vision awakens within you and all around you.

The Fresh Fruit Cleanse Physical Benefits

I believe fruit cleansing is one of the healthiest and most nutritious ways to lose weight and feel great. There are so many nutritional benefits in fruit, nature's most effective cleanser. Fruit supplies energy, antioxidants, and essential vitamins and minerals, and it is low in calories. Fruit cleansing gives your body a rest from heavier foods and allows your digestive system to detoxify, getting rid of toxins and wastes and restoring harmony and balance to your entire body.

Many people suffering from various health conditions, such as obesity, asthma, and irritable bowel syndrome, among others, believe that fasting and cleansing have been beneficial to treating their issues. There are also those who claim that cleansing helped them to overcome cancer. However, remember that if you suffer from any serious medical condition, you should consult a health care professional for guidance before beginning any type of cleanse.

Lose Weight and Feel Great

Of course, we know weight loss happens when we burn more calories than we consume. With the Fresh Fruit Cleanse, it is possible to eat lots of delicious and nutritious food while cleansing and still lose weight. Nourishing the body with healthy foods will allow you to lose weight over time and build healthy muscles and bones. Fresh fruits are high in water content and fiber, and most are low in calories. This means you can eat a lot of them, feel full, and still lose weight. If you do the Fresh Fruit Cleanse for three days or longer, you will lose weight if that's what needs to happen. If you need to put on healthy weight, that will happen, too. The most important part of sustaining weight loss after the cleanse is to continue to eat nutritiously and not resort to old habits again. The healthiest way to lose weight is to exercise and cleanse yourself of any unhealthy habits and addictions. The cleanse will help develop an appetite for nutritious foods such as fresh fruits, juices, and vegetables along with healthy proteins and whole grains.

Cleanse Your Cells

The Fresh Fruit Cleanse clears your internal system of chemicals and food additives. There are trillions of cells in the human body. These cells keep you energized, healthy, and alive, but they need a constant supply of oxygen and sufficient nourishment. Unhealthy eating, deficient nutrition, and a lack of exercise, fresh air, and sufficient rest cause cellular deterioration, which diminishes the body's resistance to disease. Because fruits contain vital substances like vitamins, minerals, phytonutrients, and antioxidants, fruit cleansing can give damaged cells the strength they need to make repairs and grow healthier. The Fresh Fruit Cleanse gives your cells the nutrition they need to improve your immune system and help fight off infections and illnesses.

Cleanse Your Colon

The health of the colon greatly affects the health of the body, including energy level, skin, and other organs. Many people believe an unhealthy colon is the cause of almost all diseases in the body. When you eat whole, raw fruit you are enjoying nature in its healthiest and purest form. Fruit is Mother Nature's most optimal cleansing food, and there is no other food like it on the planet. The fibers and pulp in fruit are the most helpful because they cleanse the waste and residue from the intestinal tract, including the colon.

The Fresh Fruit Cleanse purifies the colon and digestive tract, restores good digestion, and, by quickening the peristaltic action of the colon, helps elimination. The organs get a rest from heavier, difficult-to-digest foods, and the body can heal and repair at a cellular level. Over time, you will notice a difference in your bowel movements. If you eat three meals a day, you should eliminate three meals a day. After the Fresh Fruit Cleanse, you will find that your bowel movements are regular and healthy. Cleansing, detoxifying, and purifying the intestines, blood, and cells with the Fresh Fruit Cleanse can help your body to overcome many physical ills, clear the skin, and greatly increase your energy level.

Cleanse Your Skin

The cleansing effect of fruit rejuvenates and clears skin, and once cleansing releases toxins from the body, many skin conditions improve. Cleansing is famous for its ability to give the body and skin a more youthful tone. The skin is one of the organs of elimination; toxins and impurities in the body are released through skin pores. When the other organs of elimination in the body, such as the liver and colon, are full of toxins, the skin has to increase its own process of detoxification. This extra work placed on the skin can lead to clogged pores, blemishes, and poor texture. It takes time to undo the effects of years of unhealthy eating, but as you cleanse and eat more nutritious foods, you will see incredible changes in the health of your skin.

Many people are surprised at how good they feel and look, even after just a couple of days, as their cells are rejuvenated. Following completion of the Fresh Fruit Cleanse, it is important to maintain a diet rich in minerals and antioxidants from fruits, vegetables, green tea, silica, and B-complex vitamins from whole grains, and also to drink plenty of water. Cucumber and watermelon juice are wonderful for natural silica. Beet and carrot juice are good for cleansing the liver, which will also promote a healthier body, including better skin. Milk thistle strengthens and improves the liver, and turmeric is one of the most powerful cleansers for the liver and blood as well. When the liver is clean, the blood becomes purified and the skin clear. *You are what you eat*, so if you want to look and feel your best, eat foods that are full of energy, sunshine, and life to have the healthiest skin possible.

Mental Benefits

Focus Your Mind

If you are looking for increased clarity, focus, concentration, inspiration, and energy, the Fresh Fruit Cleanse is for you.

Cleansing with fruit helps to clear and focus the mind. When you follow a traditional diet, you spend a lot of time preparing, eating, and cleaning up. The Fresh Fruit Cleanse frees you from the time-consuming activities surrounding food. *If your mind isn't consumed with thoughts about food, where else might you focus your thoughts and energy?*

During the Fresh Fruit Cleanse, you will find you have more time to focus your energy on the things that are most important to you because you are not spending so much time focusing on food. While it's important to rest while on the Fresh Fruit Cleanse, it's also a great time to focus your mind on completing unfinished tasks and finding the inspiration to follow through on projects and goals you've put off. You will find you have the time you need to get your life back on track and to focus your mind in a positive direction. Perhaps you will finally begin the journal you've been wanting to start or you might find the time to plant a garden. Maybe you will be inspired to spend more time meditating or connecting with your family and friends, or to start a blog sharing what you are passionate about with others.

Alleviate Depression

If you are struggling with depression, the Fresh Fruit Cleanse may be a great way to lift up your spirits and clear your mind. Our choices either lift us up or weigh us down. Before you eat or drink anything, ask yourself, *how will this make me feel...heavy or light?* To feel your best physically, mentally, emotionally, and spiritually, it's important to eat light, healthy foods. By eliminating unhealthy, heavy foods from your diet, your thoughts will become clearer as you feel increased energy and vitality flowing into you. This vigor may allow you to see things more clearly and to step out of the depression and onto the path of healing and recovery. I also suggest seeking professional support if you are struggling with depression or any other kind of mental or emotional challenge.

Increase Mental Acuity

A doctor, well-known educator, and author by the name of Dr. Herbert Shelton supervised the fasting of more than 40,000 people over the course of 50 years. He found that the freer a person's body is of toxins flowing through the bloodstream, the clearer is that person's ability to think. He found that, when digesting a heavy meal, the body uses large amounts of blood and nervous energy to break down the meal. However, if that energy were not needed by the body, it could be used by the brain, dramatically improving brain function.

While this improvement in mental acuity doesn't usually happen until after a few days of cleansing or fasting, at some point during the Fresh Fruit Cleanse you will find yourself gaining greater insight into yourself and all your experiences, including what is best for your body, mind, spirit, and life. Cleansing enhances the ability to think and solve problems, and many people feel a state of euphoria as well as a deeper sense of emotional stability.

Renew Your Life

Anytime I go through the Fresh Fruit Cleanse, I'm amazed at how quickly I feel the renewing, rejuvenating, and rebalancing benefits in my body, mind, and spirit. My skin looks healthier, my body feels energized, and my mind is clearer. My spirit is uplifted, and I feel a greater sense of confidence again in myself, my vision, my purpose, and my life. I feel inspired to grow in the best way possible and to make the healthiest choices I can make.

Unleashing a Clean, Healthy Energy

The road to health is a journey. Life-lasting changes in nutritional lifestyle don't usually happen overnight. It takes time to develop healthy habits and behaviors. So, be patient with yourself and keep cleansing, year after year, and eventually you will find the inspiration to be healthy. You will develop a natural craving and desire for the choices that make you feel your best, whether in the foods you eat, the people you spend time with, or how you choose to live your life.

As you unleash a clean, healthy energy with the Fresh Fruit Cleanse, it's important to continue to care for your body, mind, and spirit with healthy foods, regular exercise (including yoga), meditation, and positive people who share a similar vi-

Youthfulness is not determined by age. It is determined by one's life force. One who possesses hope is forever young. One who continually advances is forever beautiful.

—*Daisaku Ikeda, Japanese philosopher*

sion of health and well-being. At first, you may find you haven't given up all your unhealthy habits, and some of them may still feel as if they have control over you and your life. If you commit to cleansing with the Fresh Fruit Cleanse at least once or twice a year, I believe you will find, just as I did, that you can heal from your addictions and regain control over your choices in life. Making changes is a gradual process, so let it happen over time in the way that's best for you. When you have control over your choices, then anything is possible. As you get better, the world around you becomes a better place. So I celebrate you on your journey. And I am here cheering you on. One of the spiritual teachings I have learned is that positive thinking and faith are the same thing. Think positively, and you and your life will grow better in every way.

3

The Fresh Fruit Cleanse: Different from the Rest

Cleanse While Eating Delicious Food

The best thing about the Fresh Fruit Cleanse is you get to eat healthy, delicious food and still lose weight while you are cleansing. So many cleanses are about restricting yourself from food for a long period. Although some people have had positive results from such cleanses, others find it far too difficult and depriving to go without food for so many days, not to mention having to deal with intense feelings of hunger and cravings. It isn't good to starve the cells because the body thrives on vitamins, minerals, antioxidants, healthy fats, and proteins.

Nutritional Healing with Food

Let thy food be thy medicine and thy medicine be thy food. Those words of Hippocrates are true. But realizing their truth requires transforming your lifestyle and eating habits, and sustaining those changes. Food can heal you physically, mentally, emotionally, and spiritually. We humans are meant to nourish our cells with healthy food. Many of us weren't raised on the healthiest foods. Changing eating patterns doesn't happen overnight, but it can and will happen over time with the Fresh Fruit Cleanse.

With each cleanse you will develop a taste and craving for healthy, delicious foods because you'll feel so good and enjoy what you are eating. You won't want to go back to the foods you ate before as you remember how those foods made you feel. This doesn't mean you won't want to indulge occasionally after cleansing. But you'll no longer crave unhealthy, heavy foods in the same way because you'll realize the price you pay by feeling bloated, depressed, or lethargic, or by gaining weight.

If you do eat an indulgent meal, you'll most likely eat less because your stomach will have shrunk and you'll no longer be able to eat as much. After a few days of the Fresh Fruit Cleanse you will realize how powerful and transformational healthy and nutritious food can be for your physical, mental, emotional, and spiritual well-being.

All-in-One Cleanse

While you are on the Fresh Fruit Cleanse, you can incorporate other cleansing techniques such as a parasite cleanse into your program, or other additional remedies to intensify the cleansing effects on the liver, kidney, and colon. (See "Additional Cleanses to Assist the Colon and Body" on page 183.) Even without adding these techniques, you will still be cleansing all your body's organs with the Fresh Fruit Cleanse. However, a few of the extra organ-cleansing techniques can increase the benefits of the Fresh Fruit Cleanse. With the information in this book, you can design your own cleansing program, from year to year, to make it as comprehensive as you like. Depending on your needs, you can add a salt water flush or colonic, kidney detox, liver cleanse, or parasite cleanse.

Affordable and Effective

Many food and juice cleanses are expensive. You can pay anywhere from $70 to $100 per day just for juice! When you drink only liquids during a fast, your body gets just the vitamins but not the fiber from whole foods. Fiber is essential for cleansing the digestive tract. It's beneficial to eat during a cleanse rather than go on a food fast, and fruits are the most cleansing foods you can consume because of their water and fiber content. But, again, the Fresh Fruit Cleanse is about transforming your choices and learning how to nourish your body, cells, and self, not just for three, five, or seven days but for life.

When I did the Fresh Fruit Cleanse while writing this book, I lost five pounds in five days and was never hungry, not even once. Because I was cleansing, I didn't do any rigorous exercise and practiced only gentle yoga during those days. I lost weight, felt great, and loved what I was eating, and I'm still inspired to live and eat as healthily as possible. Since completing the Fresh Fruit Cleanse, I've incorporated other non-fruit items back into my diet, like vegetables, nuts, whole grains, and healthy proteins, but I've continued to enjoy many of the recipes I ate while on the cleanse. Wait until you try the chocolate pudding. I can't believe how good it is! I never again want to eat regular chocolate pudding made with sugar and saturated fats. The recipes in this book are so flavorful and fulfilling that you probably won't feel hungry at all, but if you do, you can eat any fruit you like at any time.

There are many different cleansing regimens, but the Fresh Fruit Cleanse is my favorite by far. I have been doing it every year, about twice a year, for eight years and it only gets better, easier, and more enjoyable each time. With the wonderful recipes in this book, and others I'm sure I'll find along the way, I can see myself enjoying the Fresh Fruit Cleanse for the rest of my life. I'm so grateful for this cleanse and all the amazing, healthy, optimally nutritious, and delicious recipes in this book.

PART II

Starting the Fresh Fruit Cleanse

4

Choosing the Best Fresh Fruit Cleanse for You

How do you decide which Fresh Fruit Cleanse to do? It depends on your goals. With dishes like Chocolate Pudding, Mediterranean Spaghetti Squash, Blueberry Blast Smoothie, Tomato Basil Soup, and Avocado Salad with Green Olives, you'll enjoy cleansing, detoxifying your body, losing weight, feeling better, looking great, increasing your energy, and improving mental clarity while eating satisfying and delicious foods.

If you've been eating a lot of processed foods and a diet high in saturated fats, the all-fruit diet of the Fresh Fruit Cleanse will significantly decrease your daily caloric intake and allow you to lose weight fairly quickly. However, remember to be patient with the results you are seeking. It takes time for the body to go through the cleansing and detoxification process and for results to become visible. Stick with it because the changes will come.

Each of the Fresh Fruit Cleanse programs focuses on healing and restoring your liver, kidneys, colon, and other organs in your body. Through their nutritional and medicinal benefits, the fruits you'll be eating will help cleanse your body and clear away toxins and waste. Your body will look and feel better and you may also notice your skin beginning to glow.

Bowel movements will be regular, and you will feel increased energy once the body has had a few days to cleanse any toxins from the intestines, liver, kidneys, and cells.

Gearing Up for Your Cleanse

It is important to eat a healthy, macrobiotic diet for one or two days before and after the Fresh Fruit Cleanse, no matter which of the cleansing timelines you choose. There is no specific meal plan you need to follow in the days prior to and following any of the cleanses. However, I have laid out a sample macrobiotic menu to give you an idea of what to eat leading into and out of the Fresh Fruit Cleanse. There are many wonderful recipes to choose from in this book, so have fun exploring and experimenting with all the nutritious, delicious foods and recipes.

Allow whichever cleanse you choose to progress gradually. Also, make sure you end it consciously by giving yourself a couple of days to transition into a healthier diet. If you end the cleanse by binging on unhealthy foods, your effort and positive results will go to waste. If that does happen, forgive yourself and remember it's about progress, not perfection—but do your best to end the cleanse wisely.

Prepare Your Heart and Mind

One of the most important parts of the Fresh Fruit Cleanse is to believe you can do it, whether it's for one, three, five, or seven days—or longer. Going through the cleanse with a friend will support you tremendously when you are new to cleansing. Eventually, you'll be able to go through it on your own, though it's always good to have emotional backing. At the very least, ask your friends and loved ones to encourage and support you

The Macrobiotic Menu

Organic fresh fruits and vegetables

Whole grains

Tofu, chicken, or fish

Any recipe from Vegan Recipes for a Healthy Life (page 190) or the Fresh Fruit Cleanse Menu (page 54)

Breakfast

Hot water with lemon (honey may be used as a sweetener)

Fresh fruit

Freshly squeezed juice

Raw almonds with organic yogurt or coconut milk yogurt (try honey or agave nectar as a sweetener)

Lunch

(Make this your biggest meal)

1 serving of protein (1 serving = 1 fist-sized portion)

Tofu, fish, or skinless chicken breast steamed, poached, or baked with no oil

1 serving of whole grain, such as brown rice (1 serving = about 1 cup, cooked)

Fresh vegetables *(Eat as much as you like)*

Salad *(Eat as much as you like)*

Dressing: Vinegar and lemon with 1 teaspoon of olive oil and any natural seasonings

Snack

Fresh fruits or vegetables

Dinner

1 serving of protein

1 serving of whole grain

1 serving of a vegetable or salad (1 serving = about 1 fist-sized portion)

Dessert

Any item from Vegan Recipes for a Healthy Life (page 190) or the Fresh Fruit Cleanse Menu (page 54)

in your goals and vision of good health and well-being. As you grow healthier and positive changes unfold in your life, your family and friends may be inspired to cleanse, grow healthier, and let positive changes happen in their own lives, too.

Remember why you are inspired to go through the Fresh Fruit Cleanse, and know in your heart and mind that you can do it. Visualize yourself looking and feeling the way you hope to look and feel. See yourself making it through the one-, three-, five-, or seven-day cleansing program with success and ease. This doesn't mean you won't ever be tempted to stray from the cleansing path, but any time you feel tempted remember all the people cheering you on, including me. If you are having a weak moment, whenever you choose to cleanse, get in touch with a supportive friend who will encourage you to stay committed to the vision of health and well-being you have for yourself.

You can also journal, meditate, or do something positive for yourself anytime you feel tempted to break the cleanse. It's important to have a healthy substitute for any unhealthy behaviors as you progress on the path to well-being. If you eat something that's not on the Fresh Fruit Cleanse Menu, that doesn't mean you failed. Forgive yourself. If you are going to eat that piece of take-out pizza or some other not-so-healthy choice, you might as well enjoy it rather than feel bad or guilty. You can still recommit to healthier eating at any moment you choose. The moment to make a better choice is always *now*.

Listen to Your Body

I'm sure you have noticed that what you crave changes over the years. Most likely, the foods you craved five years ago are no longer the foods you yearn to eat now. Your appetite changes as you change, and the more you purify yourself with the Fresh

Fruit Cleanse, yoga, healthy nutrition, exercise, and positive people, the more you will be inspired to eat healthily and be well. Again, this doesn't mean you have to give up things. If you are a meat eater you might always eat meat. But you might just find you desire it less and less and that you crave fruits and vegetables more.

Sometimes, I will give my body many choices and just wait until it guides me to what it wants. I will listen to whether it's saying yes or no to a particular food. It's really interesting to see how often the mind doesn't know what the body wants. This is why it's so important to cleanse and heal yourself of any physical, mental, or emotional addictions to food, so you can be in touch with your body and know what it needs. The answer, when it comes, is obvious because it gives you a good feeling in your entire body, heart, and mind.

Cleanse Your Organs

Fruit provides the body with natural cleansing benefits. However, there are certain fruits and techniques that will help intensify the effects of whichever Fresh Fruit Cleanse timeline you choose. Each of the cleanses has been designed with specific organ-cleansing benefits to give you maximum results. Whether you choose to cleanse for one, three, five, or seven days, the focus is on awakening radiant health from the inside out in every organ and cell of your being.

Colon

If you are new to cleansing, you may find it too intense to incorporate a salt water flush into your cleansing program at first. Over time, as your diet becomes more and more refined, you will find you are able to perform this practice with greater ease. While a flush is not mandatory, it will heighten the benefits of whichever cleanse you choose. Listen to your body. If you feel it's too much for you, then don't do it. However, if your body can handle it, a salt water flush, colonic, or enema four times per year is beneficial. Flushing your digestive tract with salt water more often than that can interfere with the production of healthy bacteria in the digestive tract, causing dehydration of the bowels and dry skin.

One of my yoga teachers recommended the salt water flush to me several years ago. It's particularly powerful because it cleanses the entire intestinal tract, which colonics or enemas cannot do. Because salt water cannot be absorbed by the kidneys or blood, it moves quickly through the system cleaning out waste along the way. It also washes away impurities and toxins that can cause headaches, fatigue, and acne.

Do the salt water flush after eating the macrobiotic diet (see page 39) leading into the Fresh Fruit Cleanse. You can flush the night before you begin the cleanse or whichever day feels best during the time you are cleansing.

Salt Water Flush

32 ounces spring water

2 tablespoons sea salt

1. Drink a cup of herbal laxative tea (any brand) the night before the salt flush. Warm the water to the temperature you normally heat soup. Pour the water into a pitcher and add the sea salt, stirring and dissolving the salt in the water. Pour the salt water into a drinking container and do your best to drink all of it in 45 minutes.
2. Lie down on your right side for 30 minutes to ensure the salt water goes from your stomach to your small intestine.

(The opening to the small intestine is on the right hand side of the stomach.)

3. Give the flush 45 minutes to activate a bowel movement. There may be some cramping in the abdomen while the body processes the salt solution. Once you feel the urge of a bowel movement, use the toilet immediately. The waste that's eliminated from the body may be dark or even a black liquid.
4. Stay close to a bathroom over the next 4 hours until bowel movements subside.
5. Do the Salt Water Flush at the beginning of every Fresh Fruit Cleanse either in the morning or the night before, or anytime throughout the cleanse.

Colon-Cleansing Fruits

All fruits have a cleansing effect that benefits the liver, kidneys, and colon, but these fruits are most effective in cleansing the colon and digestive tract:

Apples
Avocados
Blackberries
Figs
Oranges
Papayas
Pears
Prunes
Raspberries
Strawberries

When to Cleanse

Although anytime of the year is a good time to cleanse, the optimal time is during seasonal changes, especially fall and spring. Cleansing in those seasons will help you build up a strong immune system to ward off wintertime flu as well as fall and springtime allergies. Cleansing in the fall will not only help you feel better physically, but it will also help you to reset emotionally and mentally for the year ahead. Fall is a time to let go of the past. Cleansing will allow you to let go of physical, mental, and emotional energy from the past year to feel revitalized, refreshed, and renewed for the year ahead.

You might wonder how to cleanse in fall when holiday parties and festivities occur from Halloween to Thanksgiving and all the way through to the first of the year. A good idea is to do a three- or five-day cleanse sometime around the fall equinox in late September or early October, and then a three-day cleanse after Thanksgiving. This will help you to feel reenergized for the rest of the holiday season—and slimmer in your clothes, too. After winter begins, plan a five- or seven-day cleanse for sometime in January to lose any unhealthy weight you gained during the holidays and to renew and revitalize yourself.

Cleansing in the spring is also wonderful. Springtime pollens can cause allergies and infections, so it's helpful to have a strong, healthy immune system. Spring is a time of renewal and rebirth, and a five- or seven-day cleanse in March or April will help you feel your best. With summer and bathing suit season on the horizon, a springtime cleanse will also help you look your best in your summer clothes.

The rest of the year, the 3-Day Reset Cleanse, anytime, will help you get back on track whenever you feel you've had one barbecue too many or eaten something you wished you hadn't.

The Big Questions

Q. Will I be limited to using only fresh fruits? Can I use any canned or dried alternatives? And what about extras like spices?

A. Every recipe in the Fresh Fruit Cleanse Menu employs fresh fruit. However, fresh fruits can be expensive, out of season, or

Tips for the Fresh Fruit Cleanse

- Read the entire book to fully prepare yourself physically, mentally, emotionally, and spiritually.
- Decide which Fresh Fruit Cleanse is best for you, depending on the time of year and your goals.
- Tell your loved ones and friends you are cleansing, and ask them for emotional and spiritual support.
- Choose your menu, and write down all of the items you will need.
- Shop for your items, choosing organic as much as possible.
- Be relaxed about the menu. You don't have to follow it strictly. You can always just eat a piece of fruit instead of preparing a meal.
- If you are going to do the salt water flush, you can do it whenever you feel like it. It doesn't have to be the night before you begin. Do it on the day that feels best for you. The salt water flush will help to enhance your cleansing efforts, but you will still feel great if you decide not to do it.
- Spend time meditating, praying, journaling, and doing healthy things for yourself like going for walks and being in nature. Write down the positive visions you would like to grow into and align with in your life.
- Practice gentle yoga, and enjoy anything that feels good, like getting a massage or reading a book.
- Envision the healthier choices you will make after the Fresh Fruit Cleanse, and see yourself eating healthily and feeling your best physically, mentally, emotionally, and spiritually.
- Forgive and love yourself and everyone else in your life, and see everyone growing well and aligning with their highest good for themselves and the planet.
- Reach out to friends, even ones you haven't communicated with in a while, on the phone or in person (rather than Facebook or other social network), and let them know you love them and care about them. Share with them how good you feel and let them know you are grateful they are in your life.
- Cry, laugh, heal, feel, and realize that you are loved and everything will be all right. When you make a spiritual effort, like cleansing, everything in life will improve.
- Reach out to a loved one for positive emotional support.

difficult to find in certain locations, so the recipes also utilize healthy, organic additions such as canned tomatoes. In recipes that need a little extra kick, I've added non-fruit super foods like spirulina, leafy greens, garlic, and flavorful, antioxidant-rich spices and herbs to help your body (and taste buds) get the most out of your Fresh Fruit Cleanse experience.

Q. Does cooking diminish the nutritional benefits of fruit?

A. When fruits are canned or dried, they can lose some enzymes and nutrients. But research has found that cooked tomatoes and carrots are much better sources of lycopene and beta-carotene than raw. This is because the heat forces plant cell walls to open, releasing phytonutrients that are stored inside, making them easier to absorb.

Q. Zucchini, eggplant, and spaghetti squash are fruit?

A. Yes. While zucchini, eggplant, cucumber, and spaghetti squash are often called vegetables, they are actually fruit. A fruit is the edible part of the plant that contains the seeds. A vegetable is the edible stems, leaves, and roots of the plants. What's wonderful about the Fresh Fruit Cleanse is it incorporates these nontraditional fruits into delicious and nutritious dishes to give you more variety in your cleansing menu and meals, instead of just the sweet counterparts we traditionally think of as fruits. Plus, these nontraditional fruits are lower in sugar so they are excellent for weight loss as well.

Q. Will I be able to resist cravings?

A. Yes…one craving at a time. This doesn't mean that desires won't arise at times, but when you cleanse regularly with the Fresh Fruit Cleanse they will no longer have control over your life. When you do get cravings, you will be able to look at them and ask yourself how that piece of cake, candy, drink, or anything else will make you feel. You don't have to deny yourself pleasure, but the only way to live with moderation is to first heal yourself of any addictions that have had control over you. As you learn about yourself, you will grow stronger and be empowered to make better choices because you will realize what has motivated you to make an unhealthy choice in the first place. Through the Fresh Fruit Cleanse, exercise, and healthy practices like yoga and meditation, and a positive community of loved ones and friends, you can and will find the strength, will, and determination to grow well and be the best you can be.

Q. Will I be hungry?

A. There are times when you might feel hungry. Remember, what's great about the Fresh Fruit Cleanse is you can eat all the fruit you want. However, it is good to pace yourself and not overindulge. Do your best to still be moderate in your eating. With the Fresh Fruit Cleanse, you will be supplying your body with the best nutrition possible. As you eat less and lighter food, your stomach will shrink a little during the Fresh Fruit Cleanse, and afterward you will not require as much food to feel full and satisfied. Remember, you can always eat fruit or prepare a delicious recipe anytime you feel hungry.

Q. What are the side effects?

A. Potential side effects include fatigue, headache, dehydration, and gastrointestinal discomfort. If you are experiencing any of these, it means your body is detoxifying and releasing toxins from the liver, kidney, colon, and cells. Continue to drink plenty of water and eat when you are hungry. Most likely, after the third day of the Fresh Fruit Cleanse, the toxins will have been released and you will begin to feel better. If you do not feel better, listen to your body and stop cleansing if necessary. The reality is when you are eating fruit, you are eating the best and healthiest foods possible. It is normal for the body to feel some discomfort when detoxifying during the Fresh Fruit Cleanse, especially if you have been living a toxic lifestyle. Continue to rest, take care of yourself, and trust you will feel better once the body has had time to cleanse and release.

Q. Is it OK to exercise?

A. While it is OK to exercise during the Fresh Fruit Cleanse, listen to your body, because it knows best. When cleansing, it's best to not push yourself too much. During the time you are cleansing it is good to be restful. Find time to meditate, write in a journal, pray, take long baths, go to the spa, get a massage, enjoy a long walk, or anything else that makes you feel replenished and renewed. If you feel like exercising, then let yourself. But you may find it feels best to do less during the days you are cleansing. Above all, always listen to your body.

Q. What happens if I don't make it through the entire cleanse?

A. If at first you don't succeed, try again. Any progress you make toward healthier choices for yourself and your life is a success. There is no destination when it comes to being healthy and well physically, mentally, emotionally, and spiritually. We can always grow healthier and make better choices for ourselves and our lives. Most importantly, don't ever give up on yourself. Let it be a journey, and celebrate each achievement you make in making better choices for your body, mind, and spirit. As you do so, you will be able to love and care for yourself and your family, friends, community, world, and planet in a better way. Wait until you feel inspired again, and when you are ready, the Fresh Fruit Cleanse will be ready for you and will help and inspire you to grow in a positive way one step at a time.

Understanding the Menu

The Fresh Fruit Cleanse Menu consists of dozens of recipes organized into categories: breakfast, smoothies, soups, snacks, salads, entrées, and desserts. Each cleanse program (lasting one, three, five, or seven days) comes with its own easy-to-follow menu plan, with different recipe options for each day of the program.

Option 1 recipes are the lowest in calories and fat, and include more fresh, uncooked fruit than the other options. Because it features lighter foods, it is an excellent choice for summer. Option 2 includes recipes that are more filling, for times when you need additional calories and fat to help nourish your body, for example, for longer cleanses of five or seven days. Option 3 consists of heartier recipes with flavors ideal for colder weather. It's perfectly OK to choose from Options 1, 2, and 3 when creating your cleansing menu for each day. Many of the recipes will give you leftovers, so this will also determine what you choose to eat during the cleanse.

When going through any of the cleansing programs, remember to listen to your body and to give yourself the fat and calories you need to feel your best. Your body knows best, so just listen to yourself and you will know what you need each step of the way. Also let yourself have fun with the menu plans and be creative. Maybe you'll even make up your own recipes. If you do, please share them with me!

Making a Shopping List

Once you've decided on your meals, make a list of everything you'll need to buy. Below is a sample shopping list—it's the list I put together for going through the 5-Day Rebalance Fresh Fruit Cleanse. I chose organic produce whenever possible.

Remember, many items such as super foods will last you long past the cleanse. The spirulina will most likely last one or two months, and the maca and raw cacao even longer. And, of course, many of the spices will last for months. Even some of the produce will keep for a couple of weeks, depending on how much you eat while you're cleansing. However, the initial cost will balance itself out over time. I hardly spend anything on groceries the week after cleansing because I have so much left-over produce that's still good.

Many of the recipes, such as Fruit Day Spaghetti, Fruit Day Chili, Tomato Basil Soup, Coconut Mango Soup, Baba Ganoush, and Avocado Salad with Green Olives, will give you leftovers. For instance, half a spaghetti squash really serves two people, and the Tomato Basil Soup makes a big pot of soup that's delicious heated up the next day.

Shopping List for 5-Day Cleanse

Fruits

3–4 pounds tomatoes
1 or 2 cucumbers
2 spaghetti squash
8 bananas
4 pears
6 ounces raspberries or blackberries
1 or 2 green peppers
2 eggplants
5 or 6 avocados
2 mangoes
5 or 6 apples
5 or 6 lemons

Dried Fruits

plantain chips or banana chips, or both (½ pound)
figs (½ pound)
dates (½ pound)

Canned Items

6 (16-ounce) cans plum tomatoes crushed or diced
1 (14-ounce) can coconut milk
3 (8-ounce) cans tomato paste

Herbs and Spices

cayenne pepper
cumin
basil
Italian seasoning spices (or any Italian seasoning mix)
chili powder
garlic
turmeric
sea salt
oregano
chili seasoning spices (or any chili seasoning mix)
onion
salt

Super Foods

spirulina (5 ounces)
raw cacao (8 ounces)
flax oil or flax seeds (16 ounces)
maca (7 ounces)
hemp seeds (8 ounces)
milk thistle (8 ounces)

Miscellaneous

fresh basil
1 (6-ounce) jar green olives or from olive bar (½ pound)
agave nectar
balsamic vinegar
garlic
1 (6-ounce) can black olives or from olive bar (½ pound)
olive oil
5 or 6 bottles filtered water

PEAK FRUIT PERIODS

	JAN	FEB	MAR	APR	MAY	JUNE	JULY	AUG	SEPT	OCT	NOV	DEC
Acorn squash									■	■	■	■
Apples	■						■	■	■	■	■	■
Apricots					■	■	■	■				
Avocados			■	■	■	■	■	■	■	■		
Bananas	■	■	■	■	■	■	■	■	■	■	■	■
Blackberries						■	■	■	■			
Blueberries					■	■	■	■	■			
Cantaloupes					■	■	■	■	■	■		
Cherries						■	■	■				
Figs							■	■	■			
Grapefruits						■	■	■	■	■		
Grapes	■	■	■		■	■	■	■	■	■	■	■
Guava	■								■	■	■	■
Honeydews					■	■	■	■	■	■		
Kiwis	■	■	■	■	■	■	■	■	■	■	■	■
Lemons	■	■	■	■	■	■	■	■	■	■	■	■
Limes				■	■	■	■	■				

PEAK FRUIT PERIODS (cont.)												
	JAN	FEB	MAR	APR	MAY	JUNE	JULY	AUG	SEPT	OCT	NOV	DEC
Mangoes			■	■	■	■	■	■	■			
Nectarines						■	■	■	■			
Oranges	■	■	■	■	■	■	■	■	■	■	■	■
Papayas	■	■	■	■	■	■	■	■	■	■	■	■
Peaches					■	■	■	■	■	■		
Pears	■	■	■	■	■	■	■	■	■	■	■	■
Pineapples			■	■	■	■	■					
Plums					■	■	■	■	■	■		
Pomegranates								■	■	■	■	■
Raspberries					■	■	■	■	■	■		
Spaghetti squash						■	■	■	■	■	■	■
Star fruits	■	■	■						■	■	■	■
Strawberries				■	■	■	■					
Summer squash	■	■	■	■	■	■	■	■	■	■	■	■
Mandarin oranges	■										■	■
Tomatoes	■	■	■	■	■	■	■	■	■	■	■	■
Watermelons					■	■	■	■				

5

The Fresh Fruit Cleanse Menu

Recipes followed by an asterisk (*) have been adapted with permission from the *Fruit Day Cookbook,* published by School of Metaphysics.

Breakfast

Chewy Breakfast Pudding*

Makes 2 servings

5 large dates, pitted
1 apple, quartered and cored
1 large frozen banana
several sections of orange, to taste

Place 2 of the pitted dates and the apple, banana, and orange in a blender, and purée into a thick pudding. Pour into a tall glass or bowl. Dice the 3 remaining dates, and stir into the pudding. Eat with a spoon.

Peachberry in a Melon Bowl*

Makes 2 servings

4 peaches, peeled and cubed
1 cup blueberries
2 small cantaloupes, halved and seeded
mint leaves, for garnish

Gently combine the peaches and berries. Spoon into the cantaloupe bowls. Garnish with mint before serving.

Spiced Pumpkin Applesauce Mix*

Makes 2 servings

1 cup applesauce
¾ cup pumpkin purée
¼ cup raisins
ground cinnamon, to taste
ground nutmeg, to taste
ground allspice, to taste

Mix all the ingredients together in a small bowl. The secret is the spices, which bring out the flavor; don't be afraid to add as much as you'd like. This dish is also great for other meals, or makes a great dessert. Eat it warm or cold.

Summer Squash Pancakes*

Makes 4 servings

1 very ripe plantain
4 large yellow summer squash
zest from 1 lime
¼ teaspoon ground cinnamon (optional)
¾ cup fresh or frozen blueberries (optional)
2 tablespoons coconut oil
blueberry jam, preserves, or compote (optional)

In a large bowl, mash the plantain well. Grate the squash into the same bowl. Add the lime zest and cinnamon, if desired. Mix to blend. If using berries, fold them in gently. Using your hands, form the mixture into patties 3 to 4 inches in diameter. Heat the oil in a skillet. Cook the patties on each side until browned, about 15 to 20 minutes. Remove and serve. Spread with blueberry jam, preserves, or compote, if desired. Or, top with raw honey and enjoy with a side of fresh fruit.

Tropical Fruit Salad

Servings vary

bananas
kiwis
mandarin oranges
pineapple
apples
fresh lemon or lime juice

Cut, dice, or get creative with the size of pieces. Add other fruits or subtract any of these as you like. Sprinkle with lemon or lime juice, toss, and serve.

Smoothies

Even if you're blending for one, don't worry. All the smoothie recipes will stay fresh in the fridge for two or three days.

Antioxidant Appleberry Blast

Makes 4 servings

1 cup apple juice
2 apples, peeled, quartered, and cored
½ cup fresh or frozen blueberries
½ cup blackberries (optional)
1 medium fresh or frozen banana
2 dates, pitted (optional)

Place all ingredients in a blender, and blend until smooth. Add more apple juice if needed.

Banana-Peach Love

Makes 4 servings

1 cup apple juice or orange juice
1 large fresh or frozen banana

2 ripe peaches, peeled, pitted, and cubed
fresh strawberries (optional)

Place all ingredients in a blender, and blend until smooth. Add more juice if needed.

Blueberry Blast Smoothie

Makes 4 servings

3 cups fresh blueberries or strawberries
2 medium bananas
1 cup young coconut water
½ cup fresh young coconut meat
1 cup ice cubes (optional)

Place all ingredients in a blender, and blend until smooth. Add more coconut water if needed.

Coconut Smoothie

Makes 2 servings

1 cup regular or light coconut milk
1 tablespoon maca powder
1 tablespoon coconut oil
1 tablespoon ground flax seeds
1 teaspoon alcohol-free vanilla extract
¼ teaspoon almond extract
¼ teaspoon stevia powder
8–10 ice cubes

Place all ingredients except the ice in a blender, and blend until smooth. Add the ice after the coconut oil is blended so the coconut oil won't clump. You may use more or less ice, depending on how cold you like the smoothie. For variety, add small amounts of raw cacao, mango, blueberries, or other fruits for a delicious twist.

Detox Blast Smoothie

Makes 4 servings

juice and pith of 1 medium lemon (remove the zest and seeds)

2 pears, quartered and cored

2 apples, quartered and cored

2–3 tablespoons flax seed oil

½ teaspoon turmeric

¼ teaspoon sea salt

cayenne pepper, to taste

3 cups filtered water

½ cup fresh or frozen raspberries or blackberries (optional)

Blend all ingredients in a blender. Try adding raspberries or blackberries to give the smoothie a refreshing twist.

Dutch Apple Smoothie*

Makes 4 servings

1 cup apple juice

1 large sweet apple, peeled, quartered, and cored

2–3 dates, pitted

1 small fresh or frozen banana

dash of ground cinnamon

Place all ingredients in a blender, and blend until smooth. Add more apple juice if needed.

Fruit Shake*

Makes 4 servings

8 ounces orange or apple juice

1 medium banana

½ cup frozen diced peaches (purchased or frozen fresh)

Put all ingredients in a blender, and blend until frothy. This is a refreshing pick-me-up.

Orange Dream

Makes 4 servings

1 cup freshly squeezed orange juice

1 large frozen banana

4 dates, pitted

1 peach, pitted (optional)

Place all ingredients in a blender, and blend until smooth. Add more orange juice if needed.

Strawberry Banana Smoothie

Makes 4 servings

3 cups fresh strawberries

2 medium frozen bananas

1 cup fresh young coconut water

2 tablespoons raw hulled hemp seeds

Place all ingredients in a blender, and blend until smooth. Add more coconut water if you like a thinner smoothie.

Green Protein Smoothie

Makes 4 servings

3 tablespoons spirulina

¼ cup raw cacao

1 tablespoon maca powder

1–2 tablespoons coconut oil

2 tablespoons hemp protein powder or raw hulled hemp seeds (optional)

2–3 tablespoons flax seed oil

2 frozen medium bananas

3 cups filtered water

3 tablespoons agave nectar

2 teaspoons milk thistle

Place all ingredients in a blender, and blend until smooth. The spirulina, raw cacao, maca powder, coconut oil, and hemp seeds have an excellent alchemy and make this incredibly healthy smoothie delicious. I'm so glad I've found the Green Protein Smoothie—I love this drink.

Snacks

Avocado Dressing*

Makes 6–8 servings

4–6 ripe medium avocados
¼ cup fresh lime juice
¼ cup fresh lemon juice
½ teaspoon powdered garlic
⅓ cup olive oil
water, as needed for consistency
salt and pepper, to taste

Place all the ingredients in a blender. Blend until smooth, and add a little more water, if desired. This dressing is great on salads or as a dip for fruits like squash or plantain chips.

(When you're not on the Fresh Fruit Cleanse, add chopped green onion or parsley for more flavor and body.)

Baba Ganoush*

Makes 6 servings

2–4 tablespoons coconut oil or avocado oil
1 large or 3 small eggplants, peeled and thinly sliced
3 teaspoons fresh lemon juice
2 cloves garlic
2 teaspoons ground cumin
salt and pepper, to taste

Heat the oil in a large skillet, and sauté the eggplant until cooked through. Place the cooked eggplant in a blender or food processor. Add the other ingredients, and blend to the desired consistency. You can keep a coarse consistency or blend into a smooth paste. Serve with plantain chips, spaghetti squash, tomatoes, or avocados.

Banana and Avocado Goodness

Makes 2–4 servings

2 medium bananas, sliced
2 medium avocados, sliced
squeeze of fresh lemon or lime juice (optional)

Mix the banana and avocado slices to enjoy the combined flavors. This delicious, nutritious snack is a healthy source of fat.

Broiled Fruit Kabobs*

Makes 1 kabob

5–6 fruits of your choice, cut into chunks (pineapples, peaches, plums, pears, blueberries, and cherries are good options)
1½ teaspoons fresh lemon juice
¼ cup fresh juice, boiled down until glazy (apple, peach, pineapple, blueberry, cherry, and grape juice are good options)

Set the oven to broil. Alternate the fruits on a skewer. Mix the fruit juice and lemon juice, and brush on the kabobs. Set the kabobs 5 inches from the heat, and broil for 1½ minutes or until light brown. Turn them over, rebrush, and broil for another 1½ minutes. Eat hot.

Plantain Chips

Makes 4 servings

1 medium plantain, very thinly sliced
avocado oil or coconut oil, as needed
salt, to taste

Try using a cheese slicer to get the plantain slices thin enough. Pour at least ¾ inch of oil in the pan over medium-high heat, and make sure the oil is hot before adding the plantain. Deep fry over medium-high heat until golden brown, about 5 to 7 minutes. Remove the chips, and lay them on paper towels. Sprinkle with salt, and feel free to experiment with spices. Plantain chips are great with Guacamole (see recipe below). You can also make chips from eggplant.

(Try making chips from parsnip or beets when you are not on the Fresh Fruit Cleanse.)

Delicious Hash Browns*

Makes 2 servings

3 tablespoons avocado or coconut oil
1 really green (unripe) plantain, grated
1 tablespoon grill seasoning (or a mixture of salt, pepper, garlic, and paprika)
Salt and pepper

Heat the oil on medium-high heat until hot. Drop the grated plantain into the oil. Flip with spatula until golden brown. Sprinkle on the grill seasoning as you turn the hash browns. Season with salt and pepper to taste. Serve hot with Fruit Day Catsup.

Fruit Day Catsup*

Makes 3 servings

½ cup tomato paste
3 tablespoons tomato sauce
⅓ tablespoon vinegar
3 drops stevia (optional)

Mix together well in a bowl and refrigerate any leftover catsup.

Guacamole*

Makes 10 servings

8–10 ripe medium avocados
2 tablespoons ground cumin

1 tablespoon garlic, minced

1 tablespoon ground coriander

¼ cup fresh lime juice

⅛ cup fresh lemon juice

2 large tomatoes, finely chopped

Scoop the flesh of all but two avocados into a blender. Add the spices and juices. Blend until smooth. Chop the remaining avocados, and mix the chunks with the tomato. Stir the chopped avocado and tomato into the blended mixture. Enjoy by itself or with other fruits.

(When you're not on the Fresh Fruit Cleanse, finely chop 1 large onion and 3 green onions or scallions, and mix them with the tomato.)

Olive Tapenade

Makes 6 servings

1 (6-ounce) can black olives

1 (5.75-ounce) jar green olives

2 cloves garlic

olive oil, as needed

sea salt, to taste

Place the olives and garlic in a food processor or blender. Add enough olive oil to help blend the mixture into a paste. Season with sea salt. Use as a dip with Plantain Chips. It's also good on spaghetti squash.

Plantain Bread*

Makes 4 servings

2 very ripe medium plantains

1 tablespoon avocado oil or coconut oil

1 teaspoon sea salt (optional)

Heat the oven to 350°F. Mash the plantains, and mix in the oil and salt, if desired. Spread thinly over an oiled baking sheet (make sure you can't see through to the pan). Bake for 15 or 20 minutes, or until firm. Flip with a spatula, and bake for another 5 to 10 minutes.

Plantain Zucchini Bread*

Makes 4 servings

1 large very ripe plantain
1 medium zucchini, grated
1 teaspoon sea salt
1 tablespoon ground cloves
1 tablespoon ground cinnamon
1 dash pumpkin pie spice and/or apple pie spice
1 tablespoon coconut or avocado oil

Heat the oven to 350°F. Mash the plantain, and combine with the grated zucchini, salt, and spices. Mix in the oil. Follow the same baking directions as for Plantain Bread.

Sautéed Eggplant

Makes 4 servings

1 medium eggplant
2–4 tablespoons coconut oil or avocado oil
sea salt, to taste

Cut the eggplant into thin ¼-inch rounds. Sauté the eggplant in a medium skillet over medium heat until lightly browned on each side. Flip the slices of eggplant several times while they brown. Season with sea salt, serve with Fruit Day Spaghetti (page 78) or as a snack, and enjoy.

Soups

Chilled Cranberry Soup

Makes 4 servings

4 cups raw cranberries (about 1 pound)
3 cups water (filtered if possible)
½–1 cup agave nectar
3 inches stick cinnamon
½ teaspoon ground cloves
2 tablespoons fresh lemon juice
1 tablespoon finely shredded orange peel (no pith)
orange peel curl or mint for garnish (optional)

In a 3-quart saucepan, combine the cranberries, water, agave, cinnamon, and cloves. Bring to a boil, and reduce heat. Simmer uncovered for about 5 minutes or until about half the cranberries have popped. Remove from heat, and stir in the lemon juice and orange peel. Cool. Cover and refrigerate for 4 to 24 hours before serving. Remove the cinnamon stick. To serve, ladle into soup bowls, and garnish with orange peel or mint, if desired.

Coconut Mango Soup

Makes 2 servings

3 cups mango, cut into chunks (from about 1 large or 2 small mangoes)
1 cup coconut milk
2 tablespoons agave nectar
black salt or sea salt
2 teaspoons coconut milk, for garnish
dry mint leaves, for garnish

Mash the mango for more texture, or blend for smoother soup, reserving chunks of mango for a garnish. Fold the coconut milk into the mashed or blended mango. Add the agave, and season with salt to taste. Garnish with mango chunks, coconut milk, and mint before serving. For an excellent breakfast pudding, modify the recipe by omitting or lessening the salt, omitting the mint, adding chia or raw hulled hemp seeds and banana chip pieces, and refrigerating overnight.

Cold Fresh Fruit Soup

Makes 8 servings

5 cups grape, apple, or cranberry juice
8 ounces pineapple juice
2 cups filtered water
¼ cup agave nectar
1 cinnamon stick
3 star anise or cloves
½ teaspoon lemon zest
½ teaspoon orange zest
¾ cup frozen mixed berries
4 cups mixed fresh seasonal fruit

Combine the fruit juices, water, agave, cinnamon stick, star anise or cloves, and lemon and orange zest in a large saucepan, and bring to a boil. Boil the "fruit stock" until it reduces by one half, then strain it. Combine the fruit stock and frozen mixed berries in small batches in a blender, and purée until smooth, or, blend all at once in a food processor. Refrigerate the mixture until cold. Arrange the seasonal fruit in soup bowls, and pour the chilled fruit mixture over top.

(When you're not on the Fresh Fruit Cleanse, try topping the soup with delicious banana cream. Blend 2 frozen bananas and ¼ cup organic vanilla yogurt.)

Cold Tomato and Cucumber Soup*

Makes 2 servings

2 tablespoons avocado oil
2 cloves garlic, minced
5 large tomatoes (about 1½ pounds), peeled and chopped

salt and pepper, to taste
2 large cucumbers, peeled, seeded, and chopped
½ cup tomato juice, plus more as needed
1½ tablespoons red wine vinegar
3 dashes Tabasco sauce
pumpkin seeds, for garnish

Heat the oil in a medium skillet over medium heat. Cook the garlic briefly, then add the tomatoes, and salt and pepper. Continue to cook, stirring occasionally, for 5 minutes. Remove from heat. Place the cucumber in a food processor or blender, and purée. Add the cooked tomato mixture and remaining ingredients. Purée until smooth, adding more tomato juice to taste. Refrigerate, and serve ice cold.

Note: To peel tomatoes easily, drop in boiling water for 3 minutes. Let cool, and the peel will slide off easily.

Fruit Day Soup*

Makes 6 servings

1 (29-ounce) can tomato sauce
3 tablespoons balsamic vinegar
3–5 tablespoons burgundy cooking wine (the alcohol cooks out)
¼ teaspoon dried sage
¼ teaspoon dried oregano
¼ teaspoon dried rosemary
1 yellow zucchini, thinly sliced
1 green zucchini, thinly sliced
1 green bell pepper, seeded and diced
1 red bell pepper, seeded and diced

Mix the tomato sauce, vinegar, wine, and herbs in a medium saucepan. Let simmer for about 15 minutes, then add the squash and bell peppers. Cook on medium heat for 35 to 45 minutes. Delicious, simple, satisfying, and nutritious.

Italian Soup*

Makes 2 servings

1 (14-ounce) can tomato soup
1–2 small tomatoes, diced
pinch of Italian seasoning
chunks of avocado or sautéed eggplant (optional)

Place the tomato soup in a medium saucepan, and add the tomato and seasoning. Warm over medium heat. Top with avocado or eggplant, if desired. Easy to make and tastes great!

Pumpkin Soup

Makes 6 servings

1 (10-pound) fresh pumpkin or 1 (29-ounce) can pumpkin purée
2–3 cloves garlic, minced
2½ cups vegetable stock
2–4 tablespoons coconut oil
sea salt, to taste
pepper, to taste
curry powder, to taste
freshly ground nutmeg, to taste
½ cup or less coconut milk (optional)

If using fresh pumpkin, bake it in the oven at 350°F until very tender. Remove from oven, let cool slightly, cut in half, and scoop out the seeds (keep them for toasting). Peel and cut into large chunks. In a large saucepan, heat the oil. Add the garlic, and sauté until tender. Add either baked pumpkin chunks or canned pumpkin to the garlic. Add enough vegetable stock to cover the pumpkin, about 2½ cups. Bring to a boil, and once boiling, remove from heat. If using canned pumpkin, add the vegetable stock for consistency and flavor. Blend until smooth in a food processor or in batches in a blender. Pour back into the pot, and heat on low until warm. Or, you can also use an immersion blender to blend everything in the pot. Season with salt, pepper, curry powder, and nutmeg.

(When you're not on the Fresh Fruit Cleanse, sauté 1 thinly sliced onion with the garlic for extra flavor. Cook until the onion is translucent. If you used fresh pumpkin, toast the pumpkin seeds in a 325°F oven for 5 minutes, sprinkle with sea salt, then enjoy as a snack.)

Rawvacado Soup

Makes 4 servings

2 cups baby spinach
1 small apple, peeled and cored
1 large or 2 small avocados
1 tablespoon olive oil
1 teaspoon capers, rinsed
½ teaspoon sea salt
½ teaspoon thyme
2 medium tomatoes, diced
cayenne pepper, to taste
freshly ground black pepper, to taste
sesame seeds, for garnish
2 tablespoons fresh lemon juice
2–4 cups water, for consistency

Blend the spinach, apple, avocados, olive oil, capers, salt, and thyme until smooth, about 2 minutes. Garnish with diced tomatoes, cayenne pepper, black pepper, and sesame seeds. Blend with water and squeeze fresh lemon juice over the top before serving. For warm soup, use hot water. So healthy and good for you, you'll glow.

(When you're not on the Fresh Fruit Cleanse, garnish with ½ green onion, chopped.)

Tomato Basil Soup

Makes 4 servings

5 large tomatoes (about 2 pounds), quartered
1 bunch fresh basil, chopped
2 cups vegetable broth
2 cloves garlic
2 teaspoons olive oil
2 tablespoons balsamic vinegar
salt and pepper, to taste
avocado chunks or sautéed eggplant, for garnish (optional)

Place all ingredients in a food processor (or do small batches in a blender), and blend until smooth, or until desired consistency is reached. This soup is delicious hot or cold. For hot soup, pour into a large saucepan, and cook on low heat for 10 minutes. Top with avocado or eggplant, if desired. This soup is packed with enzymes.

Winter Squash Soup*

Makes 6 servings

2 tablespoons avocado oil or coconut oil
2 teaspoons onion flakes
½ teaspoon onion powder
½ teaspoon celery salt
½ teaspoon celery seed
1 heaping tablespoon curry powder
4 cloves garlic, minced
4 cups apple juice
1 (14½-ounce) can diced tomatoes
1 butternut squash (about 2½ pounds), peeled, seeded, and chopped
2 firm medium bananas, sliced
2 sprigs fresh sage
½ teaspoon hot sauce
salt and pepper, to taste

In a large saucepan, heat the oil over medium heat. Add all the spices and garlic, and stir 1 minute. Add the juice, tomato, squash, banana, and sage. Bring to a boil. Reduce heat, and simmer partially covered until squash is very tender, about 20 to 30 minutes. Remove from heat. In a blender or food processor, pulse into a chunky purée. Season with hot sauce and salt and pepper.

Salads

Avocado Salad with Green Olives*

Makes 4 servings

5 medium avocados, chopped
1 green bell pepper, seeded and diced
2 medium tomatoes, diced
8 ounces green olives from an olive bar
6 ounces organic Italian dressing

Toss the fruits with the salad dressing. You can substitute freshly squeezed lemon juice or Lemon Vinaigrette (see page 200) for the Italian dressing.

California Salad*

Makes 4 servings

1 somewhat firm avocado, diced
1 cucumber, diced
1 jalapeño chile pepper, sliced into thin rings
1 (3.8-ounce) can sliced olives
juice from 1 lemon
juice from 1 lime
¼ cup olive oil

Place the avocado, cucumber, pepper, and olives in a medium bowl. In a small bowl, whisk the freshly squeezed lemon and lime juice with the olive oil. Pour onto the salad, and toss until all ingredients are coated nicely. Marinate in the refrigerator (overnight is best).

(When you're not on the Fresh Fruit Cleanse, incorporate ½ diced red onion into the salad.)

Fruit Day Salad*

Makes 4 servings

1 medium avocado, diced
1 large tomato, diced
1 small mango, diced
½ hot chile pepper, minced
juice from ¼ lime
1 clove garlic, minced
¼ teaspoon ground cumin
1 teaspoon fresh cilantro, finely chopped
salt, to taste

Place all ingredients except salt in a medium bowl, and toss well. Season with salt. Feel free to adjust amounts according to personal taste.

Grapefruit and Avocado Salad

Makes 2 servings

1 grapefruit, cut into segments and ¼ cup juice reserved
1 avocado, sliced or diced
¼ cup olive oil
¼–½ teaspoon kosher salt
1 teaspoon Dijon mustard
black pepper and black salt, to taste

Be sure to remove the membranes when segmenting the grapefruit. Arrange the grapefruit and avocado on a plate.
Place the reserved juice, olive oil, kosher salt, and mustard in a jar, and shake vigorously. If the dressing needs a little more acidity, you can add good apple cider vinegar, but do not over-

season, as pepper and salt will be added at the end. Pour the dressing over the top, and sprinkle with black salt and pepper just before serving.

(When you're not on the Fresh Fruit Cleanse, add ¼ red onion, thinly sliced.)

Ratatouille Salad*

Makes 4 servings

1 eggplant (about 1 pound), cut into ½-inch cubes or ¼-inch slices

2 medium tomatoes, chopped

1 medium zucchini, thinly sliced

1 small green bell pepper, seeded and chopped

⅓ cup chopped parsley

Basil Dressing (see below)

You can peel the eggplant or leave the skin on. Cook by either boiling or steaming until tender, about 5 to 7 minutes. Let cool. Mix the eggplant, tomato, zucchini, green pepper, and parsley. Toss the mixture with basil dressing. Cover and refrigerate at least 4 hours.

(When you're not on the Fresh Fruit Cleanse, increase the flavor by adding 1 small onion, sliced and separated into rings.)

Basil Dressing*

Makes 4 servings

⅓ cup olive oil

2 tablespoons fresh lemon juice

1 teaspoon salt

½ teaspoon dried basil

½ teaspoon dry mustard

⅛ teaspoon pepper

Place all ingredients in a tightly covered container, and shake well. Refrigerate any leftover dressing.

Entrées

Acorn Squash*

Makes 2 servings

1 acorn squash, halved and seeded

kalamata olives or capers, to taste

sun-dried tomatoes, to taste

Tabasco sauce, to taste

salt and pepper, to taste

Bake the squash halves at 375°F for 30 to 45 minutes until soft. A fork should prick through without any resistance. Scoop out the flesh onto a plate and top with the other ingredients. Add salt and pepper.

(When you're not on the Fresh Fruit Cleanse, sauté ¼ cup onion and add it with the other ingredients.)

Baba Ganoush on Spaghetti Squash

Makes 4 servings

2 tablespoons olive or avocado oil

1 large or 3 small eggplants, peeled and thinly sliced

3 teaspoons fresh lemon juice

2 cloves garlic

2 teaspoons ground cumin

salt and pepper

1 large spaghetti squash

mixed olives, to taste, for garnish

capers, to taste (optional)

sun-dried tomatoes, to taste (optional)

Heat the oil in a medium saucepan over medium-high heat. Sauté the eggplant until cooked through. Then, place the eggplant in a blender or food processor. Add the lemon juice, garlic, cumin, and salt and pepper to taste, and mix to either a coarse consistency or smooth paste. Meanwhile, cook the spaghetti squash according to directions in the Mediterranean Spaghetti Squash recipe (see page 81). Scoop out the strands onto a plate, and top with the baba ganoush (eggplant mixture). Garnish with olives, capers, and sun-dried tomatoes, if desired. You will most likely have extra baba ganoush, so enjoy it for several days. Baba ganoush is also delicious served with plantain chips.

Baked Zucchini Italianne*

Makes 4 servings

4 medium zucchini, grated
2 tablespoons coconut or avocado oil
salt and pepper
garlic powder
1 (24-ounce) jar marinara sauce
1 green bell pepper, seeded and thinly sliced into rings

Salt the grated zucchini and let it stand for about 10 minutes to draw out the liquid. When ready to cook, heat the oil in a skillet. Squeeze the liquid out of the zucchini, and sauté until tender. Add salt, pepper, and garlic powder to taste. Place the cooked zucchini in a small baking dish, and cover with marinara sauce. Top with green pepper rings. Bake uncovered in a 350°F oven for about 30 minutes. Serve immediately, topping with extra marinara sauce. I love this dish. It's so easy and so delicious.

Eggplant-Garlic Bliss*

Makes 4–6 servings

1 medium eggplant, peeled and sliced ¼ inch thick
salt, as needed
4 tablespoons coconut oil or avocado oil, divided
2 medium zucchini, sliced ¼ inch thick
3–5 cloves garlic, minced
4 ounces green olives, sliced or diced
1 medium tomato, diced

Place the eggplant slices on a sheet of foil, salting them generously to draw excess moisture and remove some of the bitterness. Allow eggplant to stand for about 10 minutes. Rinse the eggplant and wipe the excess moisture with paper towels. Dice into ¼-inch cubes. Sauté the zucchini in 2 tablespoons of oil. Set aside in a bowl. Sauté the eggplant in the remaining oil, making sure it's hot before placing the eggplant in the pan. Cook until soft. Right before it is done, add the garlic and olives. Mix the eggplant, zucchini, garlic, and olives together in a bowl, and top with the tomato.

(When you're not on the Fresh Fruit Cleanse, you'll love this dish served with a whole grain like quinoa.)

Fire and Ice Tomatoes*

Makes 2–3 servings

6 tomatoes, peeled and quartered
1 green bell pepper, seeded and diced
1 large cucumber, peeled and sliced
¾ cup balsamic or red wine vinegar
¼ cup water
1½ teaspoons mustard seed
½ teaspoon cayenne pepper
1½ teaspoons celery salt

Toss the tomato, bell pepper, and cucumber together. Boil the vinegar, water, mustard seed, cayenne pepper, and celery salt for 1 minute, then pour over the fruit mixture. Chill for at least 6 hours.

(When you're not on the Fresh Fruit Cleanse, thinly slice 1 medium onion, and toss with the tomato, pepper, and cucumber.)

Note: To peel tomatoes easily, drop in boiling water for 3 minutes. Let cool, and the peel will slide off easily.

Fried Squash*

Makes 4 servings

2 tablespoons coconut oil

1 large winter squash such as butternut, halved, seeded, peeled, and sliced ½ inch thick

salt and pepper, to taste

Heat the oil over medium-high heat. Fry the squash slices until brown on one side, about 10 minutes, then flip and fry until soft on the other side. Season with salt and pepper. Serve with fresh fruits.

Fruit Day Chili*

Makes 4 servings

2 (16-ounce) cans crushed, diced, or plum tomatoes

1 (8-ounce) can tomato paste

1 package chili seasoning mix

1 large spaghetti squash, halved lengthwise and seeded

To make the sauce, mix together the tomato and tomato paste with seasoning mix to taste. Add enough cooked spaghetti squash to make a thick chili-like stew. See Fruit Day Spaghetti (page 78) for directions on cooking the squash. The spaghetti squash is the body of the chili, taking the place of meat and beans. If you like your chili soupier, use less squash or add a little water. For thicker chili, use a little more spaghetti squash. Feel free to add additional seasonings if you'd like.

Fruit Day Hash*

Makes 4 servings

1 slightly green plantain, sliced

2–4 tablespoons avocado oil or coconut oil

1 medium sweet apple, preferably Fuji, diced

salt and pepper, to taste
2 tablespoons basil

If you like the plantain crunchy, slice it on the thin side. Cut thicker slices if you like the plantain softer and potatoey. Heat the oil in a skillet on high heat, and fry the plantain. It should take 10 to 15 minutes, depending on the thickness. Add the apple just a few minutes before the plantain is done. Cook until golden brown like fried potatoes. Add salt and pepper, and basil, my personal favorite.

(When you're not on the Fresh Fruit Cleanse, dice ½ onion. When the plantain is about halfway through cooking, add the onion to the skillet.)

Fruit Day Spaghetti

Makes 4 servings

1 large spaghetti squash, halved lengthwise and seeded
2 (16-ounce) cans plum tomatoes, crushed or diced
1 (8-ounce) can tomato paste
3–4 tablespoons Italian seasoning or basil, oregano, and rosemary
salt and pepper, to taste
diced red or green bell pepper (optional)
grated yellow summer squash (optional)
sautéed eggplant (optional)

Heat the oven to 350°F. Place the squash cut side down in a baking dish with ½ to 1 inch of water in the bottom of the dish. Bake for about 45 minutes, until the skin is dry and crackly and the flesh soft. Scraped with the tines of a fork, the flesh will easily come out in long spaghetti-like strands. While the squash is baking, place the remaining ingredients in a saucepan, and warm over low heat. If you like, add diced red or green pepper, grated yellow squash, or eggplant to give the sauce more body. Simmer, stirring frequently while the squash cooks. Place strands of spaghetti squash on a plate and spoon the sauce on top.

Garlic Tomato Slices*

Makes 2 servings

4 medium tomatoes, sliced ¼ inch thick
¼ cup olive oil
2 tablespoons red wine vinegar
⅛ teaspoon salt
3 drops Tabasco sauce
2 large cloves garlic, minced

Place the tomato in a glass or plastic dish. Put the remaining ingredients in a tightly covered container, shake well, and pour over the tomatoes. Cover and refrigerate at least 3 hours.

Greek Eggplant Stew*

Makes 6 servings

2 tablespoons avocado oil or coconut oil
4 large cloves garlic, minced or pressed
2 small eggplants or 1 large eggplant (about 1½ pounds)
salt, to taste
freshly ground black pepper, to taste
1 large (28-ounce) can diced tomatoes, drained and juice reserved
1 bay leaf
1 teaspoon dried oregano
2 tablespoons chopped parsley (optional)

Heat the oil in a skillet or large casserole dish. Sauté the garlic briefly. Add the eggplant and the salt and pepper. Cook, stirring over low heat for about 10 to 15 minutes. Add the tomato, bay leaf, and oregano. Cook over high heat, stirring often, for 20 minutes or until the eggplant is tender. Taste and adjust seasoning. Serve hot or cold, sprinkling with parsley, if desired.

(When you're not on the Fresh Fruit Cleanse, sauté 1 chopped onion with the garlic. Cook over medium heat for 2 minutes before adding the eggplant, and stir the eggplant until it's coated with onion.)

Italian "Vegetables"*

Makes 4–6 servings

1 large or 2 medium zucchinis or yellow summer squash, chopped

1 large tomato, chopped

1 small green, red, yellow, or purple pepper, seeded and chopped

12 ounces or more black olives, smashed

oregano, to taste

garlic powder, to taste

salt and pepper, to taste

Sauté the zucchini, tomato, pepper, and olives for 2 minutes or until the zucchini is soft enough. Season to taste with oregano, garlic powder, and salt and pepper. You can choose different fruits or vegetables for other colorful combinations. This dish is delicious with quinoa and other whole grains. Try seasoning it with Bragg's Liquid Aminos...so delicious and nutritious.

Lemon Herb Baked Tomatoes*

Makes 4 servings

4 tomatoes, halved and seeded

salt, to taste

basil, to taste

lemon zest, to taste

black pepper, to taste

parsley, to taste

nutmeg, to taste

Sprinkle the tomatoes with salt, and place upside down on a paper towel for 20 minutes. Heat the oven to 375°F. Mix the rest of the ingredients in a small bowl. After the tomatoes have drained, place them in a baking dish, cut side up, fill with the herb mixture, and bake 15 minutes. Remove from oven, and allow to rest 5 minutes before serving.

Mediterranean Spaghetti Squash

Makes 4 servings

1 large spaghetti squash, halved lengthwise and seeded

4 tablespoons avocado oil or coconut oil

4–5 slices medium eggplant

1 green bell pepper, seeded and sliced

1 red bell pepper, seeded and sliced

green, black, and kalamata olives, diced, to taste

capers, to taste

sun-dried tomatoes, to taste

Heat the oven to 350°F. See Fruit Day Spaghetti (page 78) for directions on baking the squash. While the squash is cooking, prepare the sauce. In a medium saucepan, heat the oil. Add the eggplant, and sauté until mostly cooked. Stir in the peppers, and continue to sauté until fully cooked. Add the olives, capers, and sun-dried tomatoes, and heat only until warm. To serve, place strands of spaghetti squash on each plate, and top with sauce.

Ratatouille*

Makes 6 servings

2–4 tablespoons avocado oil or coconut oil

1 tablespoon garlic, or to taste

2 medium eggplants, diced

2 medium zucchinis or yellow summer squash, or both, diced

2 green, red, or yellow bell peppers, diced

2 (14.5-ounce) cans no sugar added tomatoes or 5 medium fresh tomatoes, diced

1 (15-ounce) can tomato sauce

basil, to taste

oregano, to taste

salt and pepper, to taste

Heat the oil in a large saucepan. Add the garlic, and sauté until tender. Add the eggplants, squash, and peppers, and sauté until they start to become soft but still have some body. Add the tomatoes and tomato sauce. Then add the basil and oregano, and salt and pepper. Let simmer until the flavors blend.

(When you're not on the Fresh Fruit Cleanse, dice 1 medium onion. Sauté with the eggplant, squash, and peppers.)

Roasted Red Peppers with Garlic and Lime*

Makes 4 servings

4–5 large red bell peppers
3 tablespoons fresh lime juice
4 tablespoons olive oil
½ teaspoon salt
1 large clove garlic, minced
1 teaspoon liquid stevia, or to taste
freshly ground black pepper, to taste

Heat the oven to 350°F. Place the whole peppers on a baking sheet, and bake for 20 to 30 minutes, turning every 5 to 8 minutes so they will blister evenly. When they are quite soft and the skin pulls away, remove from heat and place immediately in a paper bag for 3 to 5 minutes. Remove from the bag. Discard the stems and seeds, and peel the skins with a sharp paring knife. The skins should come off easily. Cut the peppers into small cubes or strips, and place them in a medium-sized bowl. Add all other ingredients, and mix gently. Cover tightly, and refrigerate at least 12 (but preferably 24) hours before serving.

Skillet Cherry Tomatoes*

Makes 4 servings

2 tablespoons avocado oil or coconut oil
2 pounds cherry tomatoes, halved
1 clove garlic, minced

½ teaspoon salt
½ teaspoon dried dill weed

Heat the oil in a skillet. Add the tomatoes, salt, and dill, and cook over medium heat until the tomatoes are hot, about 5 minutes.

Stuffed Bell Pepper*

Makes 1 serving

1 large bell pepper, halved lengthwise and seeded
½ medium cucumber, diced
1 medium tomato, diced
1 medium avocado
lemon juice, to taste
salt and pepper, to taste

Set aside the cleaned bell pepper. Place the cucumber and tomato in a bowl. Dice a quarter of the avocado, and place it in the bowl. In another bowl, mash the remaining avocado. To the mashed avocado, add the lemon juice and salt and pepper, and mix thoroughly. Gently stir in the cucumber, tomato, and avocado. Fill the pepper with the mixture. Serve cold.

Tomato and Avocado Pizzas

Makes 2 servings

1 large tomato, thickly sliced
Italian seasoning, to taste
olive oil, to taste
1 medium avocado
sun-dried tomatoes, diced, to taste
olives, diced, to taste

Be sure the tomato slices are thick enough that they won't fall apart when you top them. Sprinkle Italian seasoning to taste on each slice, and drizzle on olive oil. Place slivers of avocado and pieces of olive and sun-dried tomato on each slice. Eat with your fingers, or cut with a knife and fork.

Yellow Squash Italian*

Makes 4 servings

2 teaspoons avocado oil or coconut oil
2 cloves garlic, chopped
4 cups sliced yellow summer squash or zucchini
1 (8-ounce) can tomato sauce
⅓ cup black olive juice
½ teaspoon dried oregano
¼ teaspoon dried tarragon
1 teaspoon basil
1 bay leaf
salt and pepper, to taste
½ cup chopped green bell pepper
¼ cup sliced black olives

Heat the avocado oil in a medium saucepan over medium heat, and sauté the garlic. Add the squash, tomato sauce, olive juice, herbs, and salt and pepper. Simmer covered for 10 minutes. Add the green pepper, and cook 5 minutes or until done. Add the olives, remove the bay leaf, and serve. This dish is great alone or served over spaghetti squash.

Zucchini and Sun-Dried Tomatoes*

Makes 4–6 servings

2–4 tablespoons avocado oil or coconut oil
1 green bell pepper, chopped
½ cup sun-dried tomatoes (about 4 ounces), chopped
3 large or 4 medium zucchini, cut in ½-inch cubes
2 fire-roasted red peppers from jar, chopped
chopped basil, to taste
chopped cilantro, to taste
salt, to taste
garlic, minced (optional)

Heat the oil in a skillet, and sauté the green pepper over medium heat. Add the tomatoes, and cook for a few minutes. Then add the zucchini, red peppers, basil, cilantro, and salt, and garlic, if using. Rather than using fire-roasted peppers from a jar, you can roast your own; see Roasted Red Peppers with Garlic and Lime on page 82 for directions.

(When you're not on the Fresh Fruit Cleanse, cut 1 small onion in large chunks, and add it in with the zucchini and red peppers.)

Desserts

Banana Bliss

Makes 1 serving

2 tablespoons cashew butter
1 medium banana
5 dates, chopped
4 teaspoons honey
lemon or lime juice, to taste

Spread the cashew butter over the banana. Sprinkle the banana with the chopped dates and drizzle the honey on top. Squeeze a little lemon or lime juice on top for a delicious twist and enjoy.

Banana Ice Cream

Makes 4 servings

3 medium bananas
¼ teaspoon ground cinnamon
¼ teaspoon ground nutmeg

Cut the bananas into small pieces so they'll freeze faster. Place in a single layer on a plate, and freeze for 1 to 2 hours. Place in a blender with the cinnamon and nutmeg, and blend until very smooth.

Banana Pudding

Makes 4 servings

1 medium ripe banana

6 dates, soaked in water for up to 30 minutes

2 to 3 peaches, pitted, or meat and water from 1 young coconut

2 teaspoons alcohol-free vanilla extract

1 teaspoon ground cinnamon (optional)

agave nectar, to taste (optional)

Blend all ingredients in a blender or food processor.

Blueberry Dessert Roll*

Makes 4 servings

1 very ripe plantain

2 very ripe bananas

1 tablespoon ground cinnamon

1 full dropper liquid stevia (optional)

2 tablespoons all-fruit blueberry, peach, or strawberry preserves

Heat the oven to 350°F. Mash the plantain and bananas with a fork or potato masher, and mix in the cinnamon and stevia, if desired. Place the mixture on a pan greased with extra virgin olive oil, and spread so that it's thin but you can't see through to the pan. Place in the oven for 15 to 20 minutes. Flip when firm, and bake for another 15 to 20 minutes. It can brown a little on the edges, but don't let it burn. Spread the fruit preserves on top, roll it up, and bake for another 5 minutes. Slice into 2 rolls.

(When you're not on the Fresh Fruit Cleanse, try a little coconut milk ice cream à la mode.)

Chocolate Pudding

Makes 2 servings

1 medium avocado

1 medium banana

¼ cup unsweetened cacao powder

Blend the ingredients until smooth, and refrigerate. Try substituting 5 to 8 pitted dates for the banana, or use dates in addition to banana. Or add agave nectar instead of dates to sweeten the pudding. Try topping with fresh raspberries, blueberries, or mangoes.

(When you're not on the Fresh Fruit Cleanse, top the pudding with chopped pistachios.)

Delicious Baked Pears in Raisin Sauce*

Makes 4 servings

½ cup apple juice

3–4 pitted dates

¼ cup raisins

6 pears, peeled, halved, and cored

Place the juice, dates, and raisins in a medium saucepan, and simmer for about 15 minutes. Then purée in a blender to create the sauce. Put the pears in a baking dish, and pour the raisin sauce over them. Bake in a 350°F oven for about 30 minutes. Serve warm.

Fruit Pie*

Makes 4–6 servings

Crust

1 pound pitted dates, chopped OR 1 pound bananas, sliced OR both combined (½ pound dates and ½ pound bananas)

Mash the fruit into a pie shell, pressing firmly. If using bananas, squeeze lemon juice over top.

Blueberry Filling

4 cups blueberries

1 tablespoon fresh lemon juice

1 tablespoon minced dates

Apple Filling

8 pie apples, grated

2 pie apples, chopped

1 tablespoon ground cinnamon

1 lemon, very thinly sliced

1 tablespoon minced dates

1 tablespoon raisins

Mixed Fruit Filling

1 cup dried figs, chopped

3 apples, chopped

2 oranges, sectioned

2 cups raisins or currants, soaked in water

Apricot Filling

2 cups dried apricots, chopped

1 tablespoon arrowroot

stevia (optional)

2 cups water or your favorite juice

Lightly cook the fruit filling of your chosen pie in water or juice. Just before it reaches a boil, add arrowroot (if making Apricot Filling), and stir until dissolved. If there is excess liquid once the fruit has softened from cooking, save it for smoothies. Drain the fruit, and pat it into the pie shell.

Fruit Pops*

Makes 4 servings

Follow the directions for any of the smoothies, and then pour the smoothie into popsicle trays. You can also pour into ice cube trays, cover with plastic wrap, and insert toothpicks. When frozen, pop the ice cube tray, and store the treats in the freezer.

Honey Baked Apples with Cinnamon

Makes 2 servings

2 large apples
2 tablespoons raisins
⅓ cup water
2–3 tablespoons agave nectar
ground cinnamon, to taste
1 teaspoon fresh lemon juice

Heat the oven to 350°F. Core the apples, but don't cut all the way through; you want to make a cavity to fill. Fill the apple cavities with raisins. Place the apples in a shallow baking dish. Combine the water, agave, and cinnamon in a saucepan, and simmer for 5 minutes. Remove from heat, and stir in the lemon juice. Pour the syrup over the apples. Bake uncovered for 45 minutes or until the apples are tender, basting occasionally. Remove from oven, and allow the apples to cool to room temperature before serving.

(When you're not on the Fresh Fruit Cleanse, combine 1 tablespoon of chopped walnuts with 1 tablespoon of raisins for the filling.)

Spiced Apples*

Servings vary

2–4 tablespoons coconut oil
fresh apples, as many as you like, sliced ¼ inch thick
pinch of ground cinnamon
pinch of ground allspice

Heat the oil in a saucepan over medium-high heat. Add the apples, and lightly brown both sides. While the apples are browning, sprinkle with cinnamon and allspice.

The School of Metaphysics

Many of the recipes in the Fresh Fruit Cleanse were contributed by the School of Metaphysics (SOM), a wonderful non-profit organization that teaches the importance of meditation, spirituality, positive thinking, and healthy living. Established in 1973, SOM was brought into the world as a place where all people of all backgrounds could come to study, learn, teach, and research the ways to live in harmony with the Universal Laws that govern creation. The *Fruit Day Cookbook* is an excellent resource full of healthy recipes contributed by students and teachers of SOM. If you would like to learn more about SOM, please visit www.som.org. I love this Matthew Marian quote from the *Fruit Day Cookbook*:

If you get trapped in feelings
gain freedom through the peelings.
Oranges, bananas
Your thoughts
you'll learn
to manage.
You'll earn stillness.

6

1-Day Fruit Blast

The School of Metaphysics suggests that its practitioners eat an all-fruit diet once a week, every week. The reason for this day of eating fruit is for people to cleanse their internal organs and cells, increase their energy by giving their bodies a rest from digestion, and to raise their consciousness about everything, not only the food they are eating, but of their own bodies, minds, and spirits and the world around them.

An all-fruit cleanse even for just a day is a powerful practice for resetting yourself in a healthy way. You will notice you have more time to meditate and reflect on what matters most in life. You can choose to eat the same fruit throughout the entire day or to vary the fruits. Either way, you will feel better and healthier. You may find there is a particular day of the week that appeals to you for cleansing, and you may prefer to cleanse on the same day each week. Or you can go through the 1-Day Fruit Blast any time you are inspired to, because any day of the week is a good day to rejuvenate yourself with an all-fruit cleanse.

I also appreciate the 1-Day Fruit Blast when I feel as if I'm coming down with something, which fortunately is very rarely. (I also stop eating cooked food and eat raw fruits and drink fruit juices.) If you think you might be catching a cold or a bug, the 1-Day Fruit Blast will help you to cleanse your body and cells and rebuild your immune system.

DAY 1 (1-DAY FRUIT BLAST)

	BREAKFAST	MORNING SNACK (OPTIONAL)	LUNCH	AFTERNOON SNACK (OPTIONAL)	DINNER	DESSERT
OPTION 1	Green Protein Smoothie or Detox Blast Smoothie	Fresh Fruit or 2–3 Dates or Figs	Tomato Basil Soup	Banana and Avocado Goodness	Fruit Day Spaghetti; Sautéed Eggplant	Chocolate Pudding
OPTION 2	Green Protein Smoothie or Detox Blast Smoothie	Tropical Fruit Salad	Baked Zucchini Italianne; California Salad	Plantain Chips; Olive Tapenade	Delicious Hash Browns; Fruit Day Catsup	Banana Ice Cream
OPTION 3 (WINTER)	Spiced Pumpkin Applesauce Mix	Dutch Apple Smoothie	Winter Squash Soup	½ or 1 Whole Avocado	Acorn Squash or Pumpkin Soup	Delicious Baked Pears in Raisin Sauce

Author's note: Detox symptoms are usually not as noticeable during the 1-Day Fruit Blast because the body doesn't go through the full cellular detoxification that it does in longer cleanses. But if you have been eating any unhealthy foods or drinking coffee regularly, you may experience a mild headache. If you notice a headache or any other detoxification side effects like mild fatigue, nausea, or diarrhea, drink some green tea, take a soothing bath, and lie down and close your eyes as you let go and allow healing to flow through your body, heart, and mind. Breathe, relax, be, and know all is well as you release the old and open up to a healthier connection with yourself.

7

3-Day Reset Cleanse

A great choice for novice cleansers, the 3-Day Reset is the easiest of all the cleanses to go through and complete. This is my favorite cleanse to do any time of the year when I feel I've been overindulgent in what I've eaten or in the choices I've made.

While weight loss may not be as significant as on the longer cleanses, you will still see some slimming results along with increased energy, a clearer mind, a lighter body, and better skin. This cleanse also offers potential cleansing of other physical and mental or emotional conditions, such as allergies, headaches, insomnia, anxiety, mental lethargy, and depression.

A good time to go through the 3-Day Reset is after festive holiday weekends, such as Memorial Day, the Fourth of July, and Labor Day to reset and rebalance yourself in every way. Rather than wait until the end of the weekend, you may prefer to start with a salt water flush on Sunday evening and begin the cleanse on Monday, finishing it on Wednesday. Create the cleansing schedule that feels best for you.

With the 3-Day Reset, you should be fine eating the macrobiotic diet for just a single day leading into and out of the cleanse—though the length of time is up to you and how your body feels.

DAY 1 (3-DAY RESET)

	BREAKFAST	MORNING SNACK (OPTIONAL)	LUNCH	AFTERNOON SNACK (OPTIONAL)	DINNER	DESSERT
OPTION 1	Green Protein Smoothie or Detox Blast Smoothie	Fresh Fruit or 2–3 Dates or Figs	Cold Tomato and Cucumber Soup or Tomato Basil Soup	Plantain Chips; Guacamole	Mediterranean Spaghetti Squash; California Salad	Banana Ice Cream
OPTION 2	Green Protein Smoothie or Detox Blast Smoothie	Tropical Fruit Salad	Lemon Herb Baked Tomatoes	Plantain Bread	Zucchini and Sun-Dried Tomatoes; Avocado Salad with Green Olives	Chocolate Pudding
OPTION 3 (WINTER)	Chewy Breakfast Pudding	Coconut Smoothie	Pumpkin Soup	Skillet Cherry Tomatoes	Greek Eggplant Stew	Honey Baked Apples with Cinnamon

Author's note: If possible, drink the Green Protein Smoothie every day during the 3-Day Reset and drink the Detox Blast Smoothie at least once to feel great in body, mind, and spirit. As you increase your vitamin and mineral intake with super foods like spirulina, maca, and raw cacao in the Green Protein Smoothie, your hunger will diminish and you will feel increasingly full and satisfied. Spaghetti squash is packed with fiber and will also make you feel full and satisfied, so it's a great choice if you crave something filling.

DAY 2 (3-DAY RESET)						
	BREAKFAST	**MORNING SNACK (OPTIONAL)**	**LUNCH**	**AFTERNOON SNACK (OPTIONAL)**	**DINNER**	**DESSERT**
OPTION 1	Green Protein Smoothie or Detox Blast Smoothie	Peachberry in a Melon Bowl	Tomato and Avocado Pizzas	Broiled Fruit Kabobs	Eggplant-Garlic Bliss; California Salad	Chocolate Pudding
OPTION 2	Coconut Smoothie	Summer Squash Pancakes	Ratatouille	Plantain Chips; Olive Tapenade	Tomato Basil Soup; Delicious Hash Browns; Fruit Day Catsup	Banana Bliss
OPTION 3 (WINTER)	Spiced Pump-kin Applesauce Mix	Fresh Fruit or 2–3 Dates or Figs	Chilled Cran-berry Soup	Banana and Avocado Goodness	Baba Ganoush on Spaghetti Squash	Spiced Apples

Author's note: As you cleanse for longer periods, you may crave unhealthy foods. Remember the mantra "this too shall pass" anytime you feel a craving. Also keep in mind you can eat a piece of fruit, plantain chips, dates, or figs anytime you need a snack. The first two days of the Fresh Fruit Cleanse are usually the hardest as you transition into an all-fruit diet. So, stay strong. As long as you have all the ingredients on hand to make your meals for the day, you'll be fine and your hunger will soon diminish as you fill up on nutritious, all-fruit dishes.

DAY 3 (3-DAY RESET)

	BREAKFAST	MORNING SNACK (OPTIONAL)	LUNCH	AFTERNOON SNACK (OPTIONAL)	DINNER	DESSERT
OPTION 1	Green Protein Smoothie or Detox Blast Smoothie	Fresh Fruit or 2–3 Dates or Figs	Coconut Mango Soup	Strawberry Banana Smoothie	Grapefruit and Avocado Salad; Fried Squash	Blueberry Dessert Roll
OPTION 2	Summer Squash Pancakes	Blueberry Blast Smoothie	Tomato Basil Soup	Fruit Shake	Zucchini and Sun-Dried Tomatoes; Fruit Day Salad	Chocolate Pudding
OPTION 3 (WINTER)	Spiced Pump-kin Applesauce Mix	Green Protein Smoothie	Delicious Hash Browns; Fruit Day Catsup	Fresh Fruit or 2–3 Dates or Figs	Fruit Day Chili	Banana Pudding

Author's note: By the third day, you may find you want lighter or heartier meals, depending on how you are adjusting to the cleanse. If you feel that you need something to fill you up, the Summer Squash Pancakes will satisfy you. The Coconut Mango Soup, served cold, is a lighter option that's also filling. It's delicious as a breakfast porridge, too. This day's menu offers lots of excellent choices to make you feel your best. Once you complete the 3-Day Reset Cleanse, you'll find you are able to cleanse for longer periods of time, when you are inspired to, with ease.

8

5-Day Rebalance Cleanse

Because the 5-Day Rebalance is a significantly longer cleanse, it's best to go through it during a time of seasonal change. That way, you can align yourself with the natural changes already unfolding. I find it best to begin this cleanse on either Monday or Tuesday and complete it on either Friday or Saturday.

The 5-Day Rebalance includes some larger meals to keep you going through the full five days. Yet, you will see greater weight loss results, as well as cleansing benefits, on this cleanse than on the shorter cleanses. You'll also have more time and energy to realign your priorities and focus on what's most important to you in life, whether that's nurturing your hobbies, interests, relationships, physical fitness, or anything else that makes you feel your best. Be sure you have time to rest during this cleanse and aren't required to engage in any strenuous physical, mental, or emotional activity.

Lead into and out of the 5-Day Rebalance with one or two days of the macrobiotic diet.

DAY 1 (5-DAY REBALANCE)

	BREAKFAST	MORNING SNACK (OPTIONAL)	LUNCH	AFTERNOON SNACK (OPTIONAL)	DINNER	DESSERT
OPTION 1	Green Protein Smoothie or Detox Blast Smoothie	Fresh Fruit or 2–3 Dates or Figs	Cold Tomato and Cucumber Soup; Avocado Salad with Green Olives	Antioxidant Appleberry Blast	Fruit Day Soup	Banana Ice Cream
OPTION 2	Green Protein Smoothie or Detox Blast Smoothie	Tropical Fruit Salad	Lemon Herb Baked Tomatoes; Fruit Day Hash	Plantain Chips; Guacamole	Baked Zucchini Italianne	Chocolate Pudding
OPTION 3 (WINTER)	Dutch Apple Smoothie	Chewy Breakfast Pudding	Pumpkin Soup	Fresh Fruit or 2–3 Dates or Figs	Fruit Day Spaghetti; Sautéed Eggplant	Spiced Apples

Author's note: It's best to drink the Green Protein Smoothie at least three times during the 5-Day Rebalance. Be sure to drink the Detox Blast Smoothie at least once during the cleanse, and twice if possible. If you find you are hungry toward the end of your first day of cleansing, try the Chocolate Pudding with blackberries—it's a luscious, filling dessert.

DAY 2 (5-DAY REBALANCE)

	BREAKFAST	MORNING SNACK (OPTIONAL)	LUNCH	AFTERNOON SNACK (OPTIONAL)	DINNER	DESSERT
OPTION 1	Green Protein Smoothie or Detox Blast Smoothie	Peachberry in a Melon Bowl	Garlic Tomato Slices; California Salad	Fresh Fruit or 2–3 Dates or Figs	Yellow Squash Italian; Fire and Ice Tomatoes	Chocolate Pudding
OPTION 2	Coconut Smoothie	Tropical Fruit Salad	Stuffed Bell Pepper; Delicious Hash Browns	Plantain Chips; Olive Tapenade	Greek Eggplant Stew; Plantain Bread	Blueberry Dessert Roll
OPTION 3 (WINTER)	Chewy Breakfast Pudding	Dutch Apple Smoothie	Winter Squash Soup	Fresh Fruit or 2–3 Dates or Figs	Fruit Day Chili	Apple or Apricot Fruit Pie

Author's note: You may find you want to start your day with a delicious, satisfying Coconut Smoothie—so filling that you may realize you aren't as hungry as you thought you'd be during the day. Remember, you don't have to eat a meal if you aren't hungry. Or you may want to substitute a snack for a meal. I love plantain chips, which are so good with Guacamole or Olive Tapenade.

DAY 3 (5-DAY REBALANCE)						
	BREAKFAST	**MORNING SNACK (OPTIONAL)**	**LUNCH**	**AFTERNOON SNACK (OPTIONAL)**	**DINNER**	**DESSERT**
OPTION 1	Green Protein Smoothie or Detox Blast Smoothie	Tropical Fruit Salad	Tomato Basil Soup	Fresh Fruit or 2–3 Dates or Figs	Roasted Red Peppers with Garlic and Lime	Blueberry Fruit Pie
OPTION 2	Banana-Peach Love	Fresh Fruit or 2–3 Dates or Figs	Baked Zucchini Italianne	Green Protein Smoothie	Mediterranean Spaghetti Squash; Fruit Day Salad	Chocolate Pudding
OPTION 3 (WINTER)	Spiced Pump-kin Applesauce Mix	Coconut Smoothie	Chilled Cran-berry Soup	Fresh Fruit or 2–3 Dates or Figs	Fried Squash; Baba Ganoush	Honey Baked Apples with Cinnamon

Author's note: Tomato Basil Soup is one of my favorite recipes, and I know you'll love it, too. It will warm your soul, feed your cells, heal your body, and enlighten your mind. Because the soup is uncooked, it's packed with vitamins, minerals, and enzymes. You can warm it slightly without affecting the enzymes. To make it even more filling, try adding chunks of avocado, pieces of sautéed eggplant, or both.

DAY 4 (5-DAY REBALANCE)						
	BREAKFAST	**MORNING SNACK (OPTIONAL)**	**LUNCH**	**AFTERNOON SNACK (OPTIONAL)**	**DINNER**	**DESSERT**
OPTION 1	Green Protein Smoothie or Detox Blast Smoothie	Fresh Fruit or 2–3 Dates or Figs	Ratatouille Salad; Basil Dressing	Plantain Chips; Guacamole	Fruit Day Soup	Banana Ice Cream
OPTION 2	Strawberry Banana Smoothie	Fresh Fruit or 2–3 Dates or Figs	Skillet Cherry Tomatoes; Fried Squash	½ or 1 Whole Avocado	Eggplant-Garlic Bliss; Plantain Zucchini Bread	Honey Baked Apples with Cinnamon
OPTION 3 (WINTER)	Dutch Apple Smoothie	Chewy Break-fast Pudding	Fruit Day Hash	Fresh Fruit or 2–3 Dates or Figs	Acorn Squash	Delicious Baked Pears in Raisin Sauce

Author's note: If you crave something a little heartier, especially in fall or winter, Acorn Squash will soothe your soul and satisfy you. Avocado makes an excellent snack anytime you want a piece of fruit that's filling but not sweet. By now, you are most likely experiencing the positive effects of the fiber-filled Fresh Fruit Cleanse: healthy and regular elimination. It's possible you are also noticing visible changes in the appearance of your skin. If a mild breakout occurs during a cleanse, it's a good sign. It means your body is detoxifying and cleansing, so give it time and you'll notice your skin becoming more youthful, vibrant, and glowing.

DAY 5 (5-DAY REBALANCE)

	BREAKFAST	MORNING SNACK (OPTIONAL)	LUNCH	AFTERNOON SNACK (OPTIONAL)	DINNER	DESSERT
OPTION 1	Green Protein Smoothie or Detox Blast Smoothie	Fresh Fruit or 2–3 Dates or Figs	Tomato and Avocado Pizzas; Fruit Day Hash	Blueberry Blast Smoothie	Zucchini and Sun-Dried Tomatoes; Avocado Salad with Green Olives	Blueberry Dessert Roll
OPTION 2	Coconut Mango Soup	Green Protein Smoothie	Delicious Hash Browns; Fruit Day Catsup; Fruit Day Salad	Fresh Fruit or 2–3 Dates or Figs	Fruit Day Spaghetti; Sautéed Eggplant	Chocolate Pudding
OPTION 3 (WINTER)	Green Protein Smoothie	Fresh Fruit or 2–3 Dates or Figs	Fruit Day Chili	Fresh Fruit or 2–3 Dates or Figs	Greek Eggplant Stew	Spiced Apples

Author's note: By now, you are feeling and looking your best, and there's a good chance you'll feel that you can keep going. If you're inspired to cleanse longer, continue for as long as you're inspired to go. At some point, you will need to break the cleanse with whole grains or steamed vegetables as you allow yourself to enjoy other foods in your life. Just remember to end the cleanse consciously, and do your best to eat something healthy and satisfying.

9

7-Day Detox Diet

The 7-Day Detox is great for more experienced cleansers—or first-time cleansers who are feeling ambitious and want to see major results.

Because you are nourishing your body with healthy food and nutrition, it's possible to work, attend to daily tasks, and exercise while on the 7-Day Detox, but it's a good idea to plan the cleanse for a time when you have the option of resting more and doing less.

I think you will find, as I do, that going through this cleanse program in fall or spring produces maximum results: weight loss, cellular detoxification, revitalizing of internal organs and digestion, cleansing of the intestinal tract, glowing skin, and increased energy, mental clarity, and focus. As you awaken your willpower, you, too, will realize that you can reach your goals, whether that's a healthier body or a dream you'd like to achieve in life.

It's best to lead into and out of the 7-Day Detox with one or two days of the macrobiotic diet.

DAY 1 (7-DAY DETOX DIET)

	BREAKFAST	MORNING SNACK (OPTIONAL)	LUNCH	AFTERNOON SNACK (OPTIONAL)	DINNER	DESSERT
OPTION 1	Green Protein Smoothie or Detox Blast Smoothie	Tropical Fruit Salad	Cold Fresh Fruit Soup	Fresh Fruit or Banana-Peach Love	Ratatouille	Chocolate Pudding
OPTION 2	Green Protein Smoothie or Detox Blast Smoothie	Fresh Fruit or 2–3 Dates or Figs	Tomato Basil Soup	Green Protein Smoothie	Baked Zucchini Italianne; Avocado Salad with Green Olives	Banana Ice Cream
OPTION 3 (WINTER)	Spiced Pumpkin Applesauce Mix	Banana-Peach Love	Fruit Day Hash; Skillet Cherry Tomatoes	Banana and Avocado Goodness	Fruit Day Spaghetti; Sautéed Eggplant	Spiced Apples

Author's note: It's best to drink the Green Protein Smoothie at least three or four times during the 7-Day Detox Diet, and the Detox Blast Smoothie at least two or three times. If you've cleansed before or the weather is warm, you may find you crave something lighter and don't desire as much food—in that case, the Cold Fresh Fruit Soup is a great choice. If you crave a heartier meal, Fruit Day Hash will fill and satisfy you so much you'll forget you're eating fruit. Spiced Apples is an excellent dessert in colder weather or just as something sweet to end your first full day of cleansing.

DAY 2 (7-DAY DETOX DIET)						
	BREAKFAST	**MORNING SNACK (OPTIONAL)**	**LUNCH**	**AFTERNOON SNACK (OPTIONAL)**	**DINNER**	**DESSERT**
OPTION 1	Green Protein Smoothie or Detox Blast Smoothie	Fresh Fruit or 2–3 Dates or Figs	Fruit Day Soup	½ or 1 Whole Avocado with Olive Tapenade	Eggplant-Garlic Bliss; Fire and Ice Tomatoes	Fruit Shake
OPTION 2	Green Protein Smoothie or Detox Blast Smoothie	Tropical Fruit Salad	Rawvacado Soup; Skillet Cherry Tomatoes	Plantain Chips with Guacamole	Roasted Red Peppers with Garlic and Lime; Fruit Day Hash	Chocolate Pudding
OPTION 3 (WINTER)	Antioxidant Appleberry Blast	Chewy Breakfast Pudding	Fruit Day Chili	Fresh Fruit or 2–3 Dates or Figs	Pumpkin Soup	Delicious Baked Pears in Raisin Sauce

Author's note: Both Fruit Day Soup and Rawvacado Soup are delicious and will give you leftovers to enjoy during this day or the following day. The Fruit Shake is a lighter option if you want something healthy, light, and sweet to end the day. Remember, you can always enjoy a smoothie anytime during the Fresh Fruit Cleanse for breakfast, lunch, dinner, snack, or dessert.

DAY 3 (7-DAY DETOX DIET)						
	BREAKFAST	**MORNING SNACK (OPTIONAL)**	**LUNCH**	**AFTERNOON SNACK (OPTIONAL)**	**DINNER**	**DESSERT**
OPTION 1	Green Protein Smoothie or Detox Blast Smoothie	Fresh Fruit or 2–3 Dates or Figs	Cold Tomato and Cucumber Soup	Blueberry Blast Smoothie	Grapefruit and Avocado Salad; Plantain Zucchini Bread	Chocolate Pudding
OPTION 2	Green Protein Smoothie or Detox Blast Smoothie	Peachberry in a Melon Bowl	Lemon Herb Baked Tomatoes; Plantain Chips; Baba Ganoush	Fresh Fruit or 2–3 Dates or Figs	Yellow Squash Italian	Blueberry Fruit Pie
OPTION 3 (WINTER)	Dutch Apple Smoothie	Fresh Fruit or 2–3 Dates or Figs	Italian Soup; Sautéed Eggplant	Fresh Fruit or 2–3 Dates or Figs	Acorn Squash	Honey Baked Apples with Cinnamon

Author's note: The Grapefruit and Avocado Salad is a really delicious blend of flavors. It's a great choice if you crave a light but filling dish in spring or summer.

DAY 4 (7-DAY DETOX DIET)

	BREAKFAST	MORNING SNACK (OPTIONAL)	LUNCH	AFTERNOON SNACK (OPTIONAL)	DINNER	DESSERT
OPTION 1	Green Protein Smoothie or Detox Blast Smoothie	Broiled Fruit Kabobs	Ratatouille Salad; Basil Dressing	Coconut Smoothie or Fresh Fruit Juice	Fruit Day Spaghetti; Avocado Salad with Green Olives	Fruit Pop
OPTION 2	Green Protein Smoothie or Detox Blast Smoothie	Tropical Fruit Salad or Fresh Fruit	Fruit Day Hash; Garlic Tomato Slices	Blueberry Blast Smoothie or Fresh Fruit Juice	Zucchini and Sun-Dried Tomatoes	Banana Pudding
OPTION 3 (WINTER)	Banana and Avocado Goodness	Banana-Peach Love	Winter Squash Soup	Fresh Fruit or 2–3 Dates or Figs	Mediterranean Spaghetti Squash	Blueberry Dessert Roll

Author's note: I love spaghetti squash, and there are so many ways to enjoy this high-fiber, nutritious alternative to pasta. Fruit Day Spaghetti and Mediterranean Spaghetti Squash are both options on this menu. Whichever you prefer, you'll have leftovers to enjoy.

DAY 5 (7-DAY DETOX DIET)

	BREAKFAST	MORNING SNACK (OPTIONAL)	LUNCH	AFTERNOON SNACK (OPTIONAL)	DINNER	DESSERT
OPTION 1	Green Protein Smoothie or Detox Blast Smoothie	Peachberry in a Melon Bowl	Lemon Herb Baked Tomatoes; California Salad	Fresh Fruit or 2–3 Dates or Figs	Roasted Red Peppers with Garlic; Fruit Day Hash	Banana Ice Cream
OPTION 2	Green Protein Smoothie or Detox Blast Smoothie	Fresh Fruit or 2–3 Dates or Figs	Stuffed Bell Pepper; Fried Squash	Plantain Chips; Guacamole	Greek Eggplant Stew; Plantain Bread	Honey Baked Apples with Cinnamon
OPTION 3 (WINTER)	Spiced Pumpkin Applesauce Mix	Banana and Avocado Goodness	Delicious Hash Browns; Fruit Day Catsup	Fresh Fruit or 2–3 Dates or Figs	Yellow Squash Italian	Blueberry Dessert Roll

Author's note: If you feel like a bigger meal today, enjoy Delicious Hash Browns with Fruit Day Catsup and add any salad, such as California Salad, for a really satisfying meal. The wonderful flavors in Yellow Squash Italian are also wonderful for dinner. You've made it this far, so keep going and you will be so glad you did. You have the power within yourself to rise above your cravings and choose what's best for yourself.

DAY 6 (7-DAY DETOX DIET)						
	BREAKFAST	**MORNING SNACK (OPTIONAL)**	**LUNCH**	**AFTERNOON SNACK (OPTIONAL)**	**DINNER**	**DESSERT**
OPTION 1	Green Protein Smoothie or Detox Blast Smoothie	Fresh Fruit or 2–3 Dates or Figs	Tomato Basil Soup	Green Protein Smoothie	Baked Zucchini Italianne	Spiced Apples
OPTION 2	Green Protein Smoothie or Detox Blast Smoothie	Tropical Fruit Salad	Fruit Day Spaghetti; Avocado Salad with Green Olives	Plantain Chips; Olive Tapenade	Delicious Hash Browns; Fruit Day Catsup; Cold Tomato and Cucumber Soup	Banana Bliss
OPTION 3 (WINTER)	Antioxidant Appleberry Blast	Chewy Breakfast Pudding	Plantain Bread; Avocado Dressing	Fresh Fruit or 2–3 Dates or Figs	Fried Squash; Skillet Cherry Tomatoes	Chocolate Pudding

Author's note: Baked Zucchini Italianne and a Blueberry Dessert Roll or Chocolate Pudding—is this cleansing or is this heaven? This is your new life of eating nutritiously and deliciously and realizing everything in your life grows well when you make choices that are best and healthiest for you.

DAY 7 (7-DAY DETOX DIET)						
	BREAKFAST	MORNING SNACK (OPTIONAL)	LUNCH	AFTERNOON SNACK (OPTIONAL)	DINNER	DESSERT
OPTION 1	Green Protein Smoothie or Detox Blast Smoothie	Fresh Fruit or 2–3 Dates or Figs	Coconut Mango Soup	Fresh Fruit or 2–3 Dates or Figs	Fruit Day Soup; Avocado Salad with Green Olives	Chocolate Pudding
OPTION 2	Summer Squash Pancakes	Green Power Smoothie	Tomato and Avocado Pizzas	Plantain Chips; Baba Ganoush	Fruit Day Spaghetti; Fruit Day Salad	Blueberry Fruit Pie
OPTION 3 (WINTER)	Dutch Apple Smoothie	Banana and Avocado Goodness	Eggplant-Garlic Bliss	Fresh Fruit or 2–3 Dates or Figs	Fruit Day Chili	Delicious Baked Pears in Raisin Sauce

Author's note: There's a chance you may be craving heartier meals today, so Summer Squash Pancakes will fill your stomach and have you feeling nourished and satisfied. Fruit Day Spaghetti for dinner and Chocolate Pudding for dessert also make excellent choices to complete your cleanse feeling healthy and strong. Even when you are not going through the Fresh Fruit Cleanse, continue to drink the Green Protein Smoothie and the Detox Blast Smoothie on a regular basis to feel and look your best. I like to drink the Green Protein Smoothie at least four times a week and the Detox Blast Smoothie once or twice a week. These two smoothies are food for your cells and heart and are sunshine for your soul.

10

The Nutritional Benefits of Fruit

Fall in Love with Fruit

Have you ever taken the time to really look at an apple or marvel at a strawberry? The various fruits are some of the most incredible and beautiful foods on the planet. Packed with vitamins, minerals, phytonutrients, and other antioxidants, they are truly among nature's greatest gifts and medicines.

The Facts of Fruit

A lot of people wonder how fruit can be good for them and help them lose weight when it contains sugar. After all, many fruits taste as sweet and indulgent as carefully crafted desserts. Well, the answer is *fructose*. Fructose is the naturally occurring sugar in fruit that's healthy for your body.

Fructose

Fructose is the primary simple sugar found naturally in fruits, fruit juices, and honey. It gives a fruit its sweet flavor. Despite its sweetness, fructose actually helps your body regulate blood sugar levels, making it much healthier than other sugars. Because sugars like sucrose and glucose are immediately absorbed

Healthy and Unhealthy Sweeteners

When it comes to sweeteners, it's important to know which ones are good for you and which are best to avoid. Here's a breakdown of some of the best-known sweeteners.

Avoid

Artificial sugar substitutes Saccharin was developed in a chemical laboratory in 1879 and has long been sold in the familiar pink packet labeled Sweet'N Low. It is also widely used in packaged foods. Because high doses of saccharin were found to cause bladder cancer in laboratory animals, the FDA requires that all products containing saccharin carry a warning label. Do you really want *that* in your body?

Other common artificial sweeteners to avoid: aspartame (NutraSweet) and sucralose (Splenda).

High fructose corn syrup (HFCS) Although high fructose corn syrup includes the word "fructose," this is definitely a sweetener to avoid. Too much sugar causes weight gain, tooth cavities, poor nutrition, and increased triglyceride levels (believed to increase the risk of heart attacks), and HFCS is the main sweetener to blame. Over the past few decades, HFCS has been added to more and more foods, including breakfast cereals, regular sodas, and packaged and processed foods like cookies, cakes, and microwavable meals because it is less expensive to produce than sugar.

Choose

Agave nectar Made from the agave plant, agave nectar tastes similar to honey but has fewer calories. Because it's a fruit sugar,

into the bloodstream, they are more likely to cause blood sugar levels to spike and then fall, which can cause a craving for unhealthy, sugar-filled foods.

Fructose is broken down into sucrose and glycogen. In order for the body to use fructose, it must first convert sucrose into glucose in the liver. Thus, blood cells cannot immediately absorb fructose when fruit is eaten, which helps to stabilize blood sugar levels and decrease hunger. In this way, fruits and it absorbs more slowly into the bloodstream, making it ideal for diabetics. It has a milder, light flavor and thinner consistency than honey, and it's an excellent sugar alternative for adding to your favorite smoothies or desserts.

Honey Raw honey is a food said to increase longevity. In addition to being a sweetener, it's full of nutrients. When honey is cooked, it loses its enzymes, so be sure to eat honey raw. Buy it from local farmer's markets or beekeepers who can verify that it's raw. Use honey to sweeten tea and smoothies and to make food more digestible.

Stevia Made from the leaf of the stevia plant, this sweetener comes in either liquid or powder form. Stevia is up to 300 times sweeter than regular sugar but with no calories. Although it doesn't have enough bulk for baking, it is ideal for sweetening drinks, cereals, and yogurt. Japanese drink manufacturers have been using stevia for over 30 years with no known ill effects.

Date sugar An excellent replacement for conventional sugar in baking, date sugar consists of finely ground dates. It contains all the fruit's nutrients and minerals. Date sugar is an excellent option for diabetics.

Xylitol Although xylitol sounds like an artificial sweetener, it's actually birch sugar—and it's good for baking. Xylitol has fewer calories than regular sugar, and it's believed to fight tooth decay. Like date sugar, xylitol is a good choice for diabetics.

vegetables help to maintain a steady blood sugar and healthy weight.

Did you know that fructose is actually sweeter than table sugar? Not only that, but the naturally occurring fructose found in fruit gives you more energy than any food with added sugar. Eating a piece of fruit in the morning actually provides greater energy than a sugary latte does.

Nutrients for Your Health

The foods we eat contain nutrients essential for good health. For optimum functioning, the body uses about 20 amino acids, several dozen sugars and fatty acids, approximately 40 vitamins, and a hundred or so minerals and trace elements. So, let's look at a few of the incredible health benefits that come from the best-known nutrients.

Antioxidants

Antioxidants are a group of substances that includes vitamins C and E, phytochemicals such as beta-carotene and related carotenoids, and the minerals selenium and manganese. While there is still insufficient evidence to know if any of these in single dosages can deliver the positive and powerful benefits the body receives when they are consumed together, science does know with near certainty that the package of these substances found in whole foods, like fruits and vegetables, can help prevent heart disease, strokes, diverticular disease, cataracts, and many other chronic illnesses. Synthetic vitamins or minerals don't do the trick. In order for Mother Nature to work her magic, food must be consumed in its whole state.

> The physician should not treat the ailment, but the patient who is suffering from it.
>
> —*Moses Maimonides*

As science continues to discover and understand the health benefits of antioxidants, new substances are being added to the list all the time, such as glutathione, coenzyme Q10, lipoic acid, phenols, polyphenols, and phytoestrogens. Phytochemicals, including flavonoids as well as lycopene found in red tomatoes, give fruits color, flavor, and natural disease resistance. These and the many other antioxidants work together as part of an elaborate network, with each substance playing a different vital role.

Antioxidants repair cell damage, boost the immune system, and provide antibacterial, anti-inflammatory, and antiviral properties. They are powerful ammunition in the war against cancer and other diseases. The reason they are so important is that they protect cells, tissues, and organs against the destructive power of oxygen. It turns out oxygen is not all good for you. The body uses oxygen reactions to burn fats and carbohydrates, which generates oxygen-based by-products called free radicals. Free radicals are molecules with unpaired electrons that seek electrons in molecules elsewhere in the body to make them whole. Often the "donors" are DNA, important functional proteins in the body, LDL cholesterol particles, and even cell membranes. The loss of electrons can alter the function of and even damage these cells and other body parts. Over time, the damage increases. Free radicals are believed to play a role in aging as well as such conditions as cancer, heart disease, arthritis, cataracts, and memory loss.

Vitamin A

Where it's found Apricot, cantaloupe, grapefruit, guava, mango, papaya, red and green peppers, tomato, watermelon, spinach, and yellow squash. (Also carrot, cayenne, and kale and other leafy vegetables.)

What it does Vitamin A is essential for healthy vision, the production of white blood cells, bone health, and regulating cell growth and differentiation. Studies show too little vitamin A can lead to a moderate increase in cancer risk.

Am I getting enough? Signs of vitamin A deficiency include insomnia, fatigue, reproductive difficulties, pneumonia, and frequent colds. Weight loss, skin disorders, and acne are also signs of a deficiency.

Carotenoids

Where they're found Most fruits, especially apricot, cantaloupe, papaya, mango, nectarine, peach, pumpkin, and winter squash. (Also most vegetables, especially beet greens, carrot, collards, kale, spinach, spirulina, sweet potato, and turnip greens.)

What they do Not only do carotenoids, like beta-carotene, act as anti-cancer agents, they also eradicate singlet oxygen—not a free radical, but a less stable form than the normal oxygen molecule that can cause damage. They also decrease the risk of cataracts, age-related macular degeneration, and heart disease. The body also converts beta-carotene into vitamin A in the liver.

Am I getting enough? Low levels of carotenoids can inhibit Vitamin A production, so signs of a carotenoid deficiency often are the same as a Vitamin A deficiency.

Vitamin C (Ascorbic Acid)

Where it's found Berries, grapefruit, guava, kiwi, mango, orange, papaya, pineapple, green and red peppers, and tomato. (Also spinach.)

What it does Vitamin C is required for at least 300 metabolic functions in the body. It helps make collagen, essential for healthy bones, ligaments, teeth, gums, blood vessels, and skin. As the body's primary water-soluble antioxidant, vitamin C defends all aqueous areas of the body by neutralizing many free radicals. It also protects brain and spinal cord cells, which are often susceptible to free radical damage. Vitamin C protects against arthrosclerosis by preventing damage to artery walls.

Am I getting enough? Signs of deficiency include weakness, spongy bleeding gums, and poor wound healing.

Vitamin E

Where it's found Avocado, blackberry, blueberry, cranberry, guava, kiwi, mango, papaya, peach, pomegranate, and raspberry. (Also mustard greens, spinach, and sunflower seeds.)

What it does Vitamin E is a powerful antioxidant that protects against the oxidation of lipids (fats) in the body. It's believed that fat oxidation leads to arthrosclerosis. As the body's primary fat-soluble antioxidant, vitamin E neutralizes free radicals in the fat-rich areas of the body. It protects cell membranes, including those of DNA, because they are made of lipids. Vitamin E enhances immune response, is thought to play a role in preventing cataracts, and may reduce the risk of coronary artery disease.

Am I getting enough? Rare deficiencies show up as mild anemia, infertility, cataracts, age spots, or loss of sex drive.

Vitamin K

Where it's found Avocado, blackberry, blueberry, kiwi, mango, pear, plum, pomegranate, raspberry, and tomato. (Also broccoli, brussels sprouts, collards, kale, mustard greens, and spinach.)

What it does Vitamin K is a fat-soluble vitamin that helps to make nearly half of the proteins needed for blood clotting. It is also essential for bone health. Research shows that women with insufficient vitamin K are twice as likely to break a hip as women who get enough.

Am I getting enough? Rare deficiencies show up as easy bruising, nosebleeds, bleeding gums, and weak and brittle bones.

B6

Where it's found Avocado, banana, date, grape, guava, mango, pineapple, pomegranate, and watermelon. (Also beans, broccoli, cabbage, meat, nuts, and spirulina.)

What it does Vitamin B6 is a group of six related compounds that are primarily involved in breaking down amino acids, the building blocks used to make proteins. B6 is believed to be effective in treating PMS. B6 also helps to convert tryptophan into serotonin, the important chemical messenger used by the brain and nervous system. As a result, B6 has been used as a treatment for depression, attention deficit disorder, and other serotonin-related problems, though no solid evidence proves it's effective.

Am I getting enough? A deficiency shows up as anemia, depression, and skin inflammation (dermatitis).

B12

Where it's found Spirulina, kelp, blue-green algae, miso, tempeh, tofu. (Also calf's liver, snapper, venison, scallops, shrimp, salmon, beef, eggs.)

What it does Vitamin B12 is known to be effective in supporting the production of red blood cells and treating anemia. It also helps nerve cells to develop properly and helps cells metabolize protein, carbohydrates, and fat. It's also believed to be beneficial in treating alcoholism, arthritis, cancer, celiac disease, fatigue, leukemia, lupus, and multiple sclerosis.

Am I getting enough? Signs of deficiency show up as decreased blood clotting, depression, difficulty swallowing, fatigue, heart palpitations, menstrual problems, nervousness, numbness in feet, red tongue, paleness, tingling in feet, and weak pulse.

Folic Acid (Folate)

Where it's found Avocado, banana, bell pepper, cantaloupe, grapefruit, eggplant, orange, papaya, strawberry, raspberry, tomato, summer squash, and winter squash. (Also asparagus, mustard greens, romaine, and spinach.)

What it does Considered to be a brain food, folate is also needed for energy production and the formation of red blood cells. It helps to strengthen the immune system by aiding in the healthy and proper formation of white blood cells, and is important for healthy cell division and replication. Along with vitamins B6 and B12, folic acid is also believed to be particularly powerful in reducing heart disease and cancer.

Am I getting enough? Signs of deficiency include anemia, apathy, digestive problems, fatigue, weakness, premature graying hair, insomnia, difficulty breathing, memory problems, and birth defects.

Choline

Where it's found Apricot, avocado, banana, blackberry, blueberry, date, orange, pear, pineapple, plum, and raspberry. (Also cauliflower, flax seeds, lentils, oats, potato, and sesame seeds.)

What it does An essential nutrient in the B vitamin family, choline helps to transmit nerve impulses from the brain through the central nervous system. It's also vital for gall bladder regulation, liver function, lecithin formation, hormone production, and minimizing fat in the liver.

Am I getting enough? Signs of deficiency include fatty buildup in the liver, an inability to digest fats, kidney and liver impairment, cardiac symptoms, gastric ulcers, and high blood pressure.

Calcium

Where it's found Blackberry, date, fig, grapefruit, orange, pomegranate, and prune. (Also almonds and other nuts, broccoli, dairy foods, dark green leafy vegetables, seafood, and spirulina.)

What it does Calcium is vital for healthy bones, teeth, and gums. It also helps to maintain a regular heartbeat, transmit nerve impulses, lower cholesterol, and prevent cardiovascular disease.

Am I getting enough? Signs of deficiency include muscle spasms or cramps, and weak and brittle bones.

Manganese

Where it's found Avocado, banana, bell pepper, berries, eggplant, fig, grapefruit, guava, kiwi, pineapple, pomegranate, and tomato. (Also nuts, romaine lettuce, spinach, and spirulina.)

What it does Small amounts of manganese are important for protein and fat metabolism, a healthy immune system, healthy nerves, and blood sugar regulation. Manganese is also needed for the formation of cartilage and joint fluid, and it aids in the formation of mother's milk.

Am I getting enough? Deficiencies are extremely rare, but could lead to atherosclerosis, eye problems, hearing disorders, hypertension, high cholesterol, and memory loss.

Magnesium

Where it's found Avocado, banana, blackberry, date, guava, kiwi, passion fruit, pomegranate, raspberry, strawberry, summer squash, tomato, and watermelon. Raw cacao is one of the most magnesium-rich foods on the planet, and spirulina is another good source.

What it does Magnesium is essential for strengthening bones, making new cells, activating B vitamins, relaxing nerves and muscles, clotting blood, building DNA and proteins, and releasing the energy in food.

Am I getting enough? A deficiency shows up as fatigue, nervousness, insomnia, heart problems, high blood pressure, weak and brittle bones, and muscle weakness and cramps.

Potassium

Where it's found Avocado, banana, cherry, date, grapefruit, guava, kiwi, papaya, passion fruit, pomegranate, and watermelon. (Also almond, spirulina, and Swiss chard.)

What it does Potassium plays a role in healthy heart function. It can lower blood pressure and reduce the chances of stroke. It helps maintain normal fluid balance in the body.

Am I getting enough? Too little potassium can make you feel tired, trigger extra heartbeats, and cause muscle cramps or pain.

Selenium

Where it's found Banana, date, guava, mango, passion fruit, pomegranate, and watermelon. (Also asparagus, brussels sprouts, and spirulina.)

What it does Selenium is a vital antioxidant, especially when combined with vitamin E. Its principal function is to inhibit the oxidation of lipids (fats). Selenium protects the immune system by preventing the formation of free radicals. It's also believed to help prevent the formation of certain types of tumors.

Am I getting enough? Signs of deficiency include exhaustion, high cholesterol, infections, and sterility. Too little selenium has also been linked to cancer and heart disease, but too much selenium can be detrimental, causing arthritis, brittle nails, hair loss, and liver and kidney dysfunction.

11

Fruits by the Numbers

All fruits are healthy and nutritious, but some have less sugar than others. The following fruits are listed in order of sugar content, from lowest to highest. The first grouping includes fruits lowest in sugar, and the second grouping lists fruits low to medium in sugar.

Fruits Lowest in Sugar

Avocado

Very low in sugars, avocado is also one of nature's healthiest forms of naturally occurring fat. The omega-3 fatty acids in avocados are believed to lower cholesterol. The fruit is a rich source of vitamin E, which helps to protect against many diseases, and of glutathione, an antioxidant that researchers believe prevents cancer and heart disease and slows down aging. Researchers have also found that certain nutrients are absorbed better by the body when eaten with an avocado. This is a wonderful fruit for adding vitamins, minerals, and healthy fats to your diet—and even if you want to lose weight, you can still enjoy avocados in moderation.

Nutrition

One medium-sized avocado contains cholesterol-lowering beta-sitosterol as well as oleic acid, shown in numerous studies to prevent breast cancer:

NUTRIENT	AMOUNT	% DAILY VALUE
Monounsaturated Fat	29 g	--
Vitamin E	4.16 mg	19%
Vitamin C	20 mg	33%
Fiber	9.2 g	36%
ORAC Value: 1,933	Sugars: 1.0 g	

How to Choose

Pick an avocado that is slightly soft to the touch but has no cracks or sunken spots. Look for fruit that has a little bit of a neck at the top instead of being just rounded. Avocados can ripen at home and, once ripened, will usually last in the refrigerator for a week. You'll find many delicious avocado recipes in this book, but the fruit is also wonderful simply cut in half and eaten with a spoon, served with tomatoes and hummus, or made into guacamole.

Lime

The vitamins and minerals in limes, including vitamins A and C, make them excellent for alleviating arthritis, liver ailments, and constipation. The citric acid in limes is a fat burner and great for weight loss. The fruit also contains antioxidant flavonoid compounds, which have been shown to stop cell division in cancer cells. Compounds in citrus fruits called limonoids have been shown to help fight cancer of the mouth, skin, breast, stomach, colon, and lung. Lime is good for the skin and can be rubbed on to get rid of dead cells and heal rashes and bruises, and added to bathwater for a refreshing soak.

Nutrition

Limes contain a high amount of antioxidant superpower vitamin C:

NUTRIENT	AMOUNT	% DAILY VALUE
Vitamin C	19.5 mg	33%
Calcium	22 mg	2.2%
Beta-carotene	20 mcg	--
Magnesium	4 mg	10%
Choline	3.4 mg	--
Fiber	1.9 g	8%
ORAC Value: 823	Sugars: 1.1 g	

The ORAC Scale

Oxidative stress is thought to be a key factor in many chronic and degenerative diseases. In Chapter 10, I talked about the destructive power of oxygen, in the form of free radicals. External factors such as pollutants in the air, water, and food supply can cause the formation of free radicals, but they are also produced during normal metabolism and cell function. The human body has various ways to eliminate free radicals from the body, but it needs the help of antioxidants, including potent vitamins and minerals, to strengthen cells.

The ORAC (Oxygen Radical Absorbance Capacity) scale is one of the most reliable methods for measuring antioxidant capacity. The scale tells us which foods are highest in antioxidants. The higher the ORAC number, the greater the ability of a food to minimize the effects of free radicals. Some essential oils and spices like rose, cumin, ginger, clary sage, and myrrh are incredibly high on the ORAC scale, with numbers ranging anywhere from 82,000 to 380,000. This is why it's so important to include super foods like raw chocolate (80,933) and spirulina (61,900), because no fruit or vegetable has an ORAC value higher than 10,000.

How to Choose

Look for bright green fruit without any bruising or scarring and choose limes that are heavy for their size. Be sure to smell the lime to make sure it is fragrant and fresh. It's best to keep limes at room temperature for ripening, but, once ripe, limes can be stored in the fridge to prolong their freshness. Store any unused cut limes in the refrigerator to preserve freshness as well.

Lemon

Lemon's detoxifying effect on your liver has remarkable results for your skin. The liver detoxifies the blood, so the purer your liver, the better your skin. Rubbing lemon juice on your face is also beneficial in treating fine lines and wrinkles. You'll be amazed at how good drinking the juice of a whole lemon a few times a week, blended into your favorite citrus drinks like the Detox Blast Smoothie, will make you look and feel. By providing healthy antioxidants to your body, the vitamin C in lemon also helps to boost your immune system.

Nutrition

Lemons contain an amazing amount of vitamin C and bone-fortifying calcium:

NUTRIENT	AMOUNT	% DAILY VALUE
Vitamin C	44.5 mg	74%
Calcium	22 mg	2.2%
Potassium	116 mg	3.3%
Magnesium	7 mg	1.8%
Fiber	2.4 g	1%
ORAC Value: 1,225	Sugars: 2.1 g	

How to Choose

It's best to pick lemons with thin skins because they have more flesh and are juicier than thick-skinned lemons. Avoid lemons that are wrinkly or soft or have hard patches on their skin. Choose lemons that are heavy for their size and that are fully yellow in color with peels that have a finely grained texture.

Bell Pepper

Bell peppers of all colors contain some of the richest antioxidants available, such as vitamins A and C. Red bell peppers contain lycopene, a carotenoid that is believed to reduce the risk of prostate, cervical, bladder, and pancreatic cancers. The fiber in bell peppers is also believed by many to be beneficial in reducing the risk of colon cancer.

Nutrition

Just one medium-sized bell pepper contains rich amounts of calcium and potassium:

NUTRIENT	AMOUNT	% DAILY VALUE
Calcium	12 mg	1.2%
Potassium	208 mg	6%
Vitamin C	96 mg	160%
Vitamin A	440 IU	9%
Beta-carotene	248 mcg	--
Vitamin K	8.8 mcg	11%
Fiber	2 g	8%
ORAC Value: 923 Sugars: 2.8 g		

How to Choose

Conventionally grown bell peppers tend to contain pesticide residue, so it's wise to buy organic. Look for peppers with a deep, bright color, smooth skin, and no bruises. Bell peppers are best stored in the refrigerator and will usually last about a week. If freezing peppers, be sure to freeze them whole to maintain their full nutritional benefits and flavor.

Summer Squash

Contrary to its name, summer squash, which includes zucchini and yellow squash, is now available year round. A relative of the melon and cucumber family, summer squash comes in many different varieties varying in shape, color, size, and flavor. The entire squash is edible including its flesh, seeds, and skin. While not as potent as other root vegetables like garlic or onion, summer squash is believed to have anti-cancer benefits. It is are also an excellent source of manganese and vitamin C and a good source of magnesium, vitamin A, fiber, potassium, and folate. Magnesium has been shown to help reduce the risk of heart attack and stroke, and studies show many of the other nutrients are helpful in preventing artherosclerosis. Fiber has been shown to lower cholesterol. So summer squash are beneficial in summer and all year round.

Nutrition

A cup of summer squash is low in calories and fat, and provides good amounts of vitamin C and fiber:

NUTRIENT	AMOUNT	% DAILY VALUE
Fat	0.4 g	--
Calcium	20 mg	2%
Vitamin C	22.2 mg	33%
Potassium	324 mg	9%
Folate	30 mcg	7.5%
Vitamin A	248 IU	5%
Iron	0.46 mg	2.5%
Manganese	0.219	11%
Fiber	1.2 g	5%
ORAC Value: 180	Sugars: 3.1 g	

How to Choose

When picking your squash, look for ones that are heavy for their size with shiny skin and no blemishes. They are delicate, so handle with care. Store the squash, unwashed, in a plastic bag in the refrigerator and it will keep for about seven days. When ready to use, wash thoroughly and cut off both ends.

Tomato

The health benefits of tomatoes have been studied extensively because of lycopene, the cancer-fighting carotenoid in red tomatoes. Lycopene is believed to be protective against colorectal, prostate, breast, lung, and pancreatic cancers. It is best to eat tomatoes containing this pigment with foods that are high in fat, like avocados and olive oil because carotenoids are fat soluble and best absorbed into the body along with fats. Tomatoes come in other colors, too, including yellow, green, purple, orange, and brown. For the greatest benefit, look for products containing the whole tomato, including their peels. And, when eating catsup, definitely go for the organic brands because they have three times the amount of cancer-fighting carotenoids as nonorganic brands.

Nutrition

Tomatoes contain an incredible amount of lycopene, and a meduim-sized one is just 91 calories.

NUTRIENT	AMOUNT	% DAILY VALUE
Potassium	292 mg	8%
Vitamin C	16.9 mg	28%
Magnesium	14 mg	4%
Vitamin A	1,025 IU	21%
Lycopene	3,165 mcg	--
Fiber	1.5 g	6%
ORAC Value: 367 Sugars: 3.2 g		

How to Choose

To get the maximum health benefits of lycopene, pick tomatoes that are the deepest shade of red. Any tomato should be very slightly soft to the touch and have no bruises or punctures. A ripe tomato has a sweet fragrance, so be sure to smell the fruit.

Apricot

Wonderfully sweet and tangy, apricots can make your mouth water just thinking of them. Small and golden orange with velvety skin, they are an excellent source of beta-carotene, lycopene, and vitamins A and C. They also contain potassium, which is great for stamina.

Nutrition

Apricots contain only 17 calories each:

NUTRIENT	AMOUNT	% DAILY VALUE
Fat	0.14 g	--
Beta-carotene	383 mcg	--
Potassium	91 mg	--
Vitamin C	3.5 mg	6%
Vitamin A	674 IU	13%
Fiber	0.7 g	3%
ORAC Value: 1,115	Sugars: 3.2 g	

How to Choose

Pick apricots with a rich orange color rather than pale orange or yellow. Apricots should be slightly soft to the touch with smooth, unbruised skin. Ripe apricots have a sweet fragrance. The best time to eat the fruit is when it's fresh and in season; the rest of the year you're better off eating dried apricots. Any apricots you see fresh in winter were picked underripe, so they may have been shipped a long distance.

Spaghetti Squash

Although it's not a high-fat food, spaghetti squash does contain omega-3 fatty acids, which are excellent for cellular health. With its spaghetti-like strands, this winter squash makes a delicious, nutritious, and low-calorie substitute for pasta. Top the strands with marinara sauce, chili sauce, or any other creative concoction for an amazing dish.

Nutrition

Full of omega-3 fatty acids, 1 cup of cooked spaghetti squash is only 40 calories:

NUTRIENT	AMOUNT	% DAILY VALUE
Vitamin C	5.4 mg	9%
Potassium	180 mg	5%
Magnesium	17 mg	4%
Fiber	2 g	8%
ORAC Value: 396	Sugars: 3.0 g	

How to Choose

While it's not essential to buy organic, I think an organically grown spaghetti squash is much more flavorful than a conventionally grown one. Choose a squash that's heavy for its size with firm, shiny, pale yellow, or ivory skin. If the squash is green or white, it's not ripe.

Guava

Common in tropical countries, guava is a delicious fruit with a ton of nutritional benefits. Many Asian cultures believe that a couple of guavas each season keep the doctor away for the year, in the same way that Americans often assert that an apple a day keeps the doctor away. Guavas have small, hard seeds covering the pulp, which is often said to taste like a combination of strawberries and pears. The fruit is incredibly rich in vitamin C, (five times the amount of an orange) and contains carotenoids and many other antioxidants. Guava flesh may be red, pink, yellow, or white. Red-fleshed fruit is a great source of lycopene.

Nutrition

One medium (55-gram) guava contains a whopping 125 mg of vitamin C and only 37 calories:

NUTRIENT	AMOUNT	% DAILY VALUE
Fat	0.5 g	--
Vitamin C	125 mg	208%
Fiber	3 g	12%
Folate	27 mcg	7%
Vitamin A	343 IU	7%
Fiber	3 g	12%
ORAC Value: 1,990	Sugars: 5.0 g	

How to Choose

Ripe guavas are fragrant, with skin that is yellow, light green, or maroon and flesh ranging from white to maroon. The fruit should be slightly soft to the touch when ready to eat, but guavas sold in markets are often firmer and should be ripened at room temperature. Once ripe, guavas should be refrigerated and used within two days. Sweet or low-acid guavas are best eaten raw; highly acidic guavas are best for cooking.

Coconut Water

Said to be the fluid of life, coconut water has the same electrolytic balance as blood. It was even used in World War II to give emergency plasma transfusions to wounded soldiers in the Pacific. It contains more potassium than bananas or sports drinks, is healthier than milk, and has no cholesterol. One of the best hydrating fluids, coconut water will energize, refresh, and renew your cells and skin. Just crack open the top of the coconut, grab a straw, and enjoy. Then split in half to scoop out the edible flesh for a delicious and nutritious treat. Check out this site for great instructions on how to open a young coconut: www.rawguru.com/openyoungcoconut.html.

Nutrition

The water from one medium-sized coconut contains a very high amount of potassium:

NUTRIENT	AMOUNT	% DAILY VALUE
Fat	0.41 g	--
Calcium	49 mg	5%
Potassium	515 mg	15%
Sodium	216 mg	9%
Vitamin C	4.9 mg	8%
Fiber	2.3 g	9%
ORAC Value: --	Sugars: 5.4 g	

How to Choose

Although you can buy coconut water in cans, it's best to drink it fresh from a young coconut because the canned water is pasteurized. Nowadays, many Asian supermarkets and natural grocery stores carry young coconuts, so they are easy to find. Look for fruit that is labeled "young coconut"—you don't want a mature coconut. Pick one that is heavy for its size and shake it. The coconut should be so full of liquid that you don't hear any sloshing sounds. The sides and top (often shaped into a point) should be firm, though the bottom can have a little give.

Raspberry

Packed with fiber and antioxidants, raspberries are among the healthiest and most nutritious fruits. They are an excellent source of manganese and vitamin C, which help to protect the body's tissues and cells from oxygen-related damage. Like blackberries, they contain a powerful antioxidant called ellagic acid, which neutralizes free radicals and helps to prevent damage to cell membranes. Raspberries have almost 50 percent higher antioxidant activity than strawberries. With a low impact on blood sugar, they reduce cravings and are a delicious and nutritionally beneficial addition to your diet. Raspberries can be frozen and are excellent for adding to your favorite smoothie or snack.

Nutrition

Raspberries are high in fiber and antioxidants, while delivering just 64 calories in a 1 cup serving:

NUTRIENT	AMOUNT	% DAILY VALUE
Fat	0.8 g	1%
Calcium	31 mg	3%
Vitamin C	32 mg	53%
Potassium	186 mg	53%
Fiber	8 g	3%
ORAC Value: 4,882	Sugars: 5.5 g	

How to Choose

The most common raspberries are red, but they come in other colors, including black, purple, yellow, and white. Look for berries that are firm, shiny, and vibrantly colored. Dull or wrinkled berries are often past their prime. Because raspberries are highly perishable, it's best to purchase them no more than a couple of days beforehand and refrigerate them until use. If you find any moldy berries in the basket, remove them before storage.

Plum

Related to peaches and cherries, plums are juicy, tart, and sweet at the same time, and full of fiber and cancer-fighting antioxidants. The many plum varieties include types with red, purple, yellow, green, or blue-black fruit. Plums have been shown to increase the absorption of iron, which promotes good blood circulation and healthy tissue growth. Both plums and prunes (dried plums) are full of phytonutrients.

Nutrition

Plums are high in fiber and low in calories:

NUTRIENT	AMOUNT	% DAILY VALUE
Fat	0.18 g	--
Potassium	104 mg	3%
Vitamin C	6.3 mg	10%
Beta-carotene	125 mcg	--
Lutein	48 mcg	--
Vitamin A	228 IU	5%
Vitamin K	4.2 mcg	5%
ORAC Value: 6,259	Sugars: 6.4 g	

How to Choose

Ripe plums should be free of any bruises or other damage to the skin, and slightly soft to the touch, though somewhat firm at the tip. Although plums can be bought underripe and ripened at home, they may not develop full flavor or texture. Ripe plums do not last very long, but they can be stored in the refrigerator to help extend their life.

Blackberry

Incredibly nutritious, sweet-tart blackberries are rich in vitamins, minerals, fiber, and antioxidants. Just 1 cup contains 50 percent of the daily recommended amount of vitamin C. Like all other berries, they contain ellagic acid, which, in addition to its role in neutralizing free radicals and helping to prevent damage to cell membranes, is believed to protect the skin from ultraviolet damage. New research is also finding ellagic acid may help to repair already existing sun damage. Blackberries are a wonderful addition to any smoothie or as a snack.

Nutrition

Blackberries are low in fat and contain only 62 calories per cup:

NUTRIENT	AMOUNT	% DAILY VALUE
Fat	0.7 g	1%
Vitamin C	30 g	50%
Omega-3 fatty acids	135 mg	--
Potassium	233 mg	7%
Magnesium	29 mg	7%
Vitamin K	28.5 mcg	36%
Fiber	7.6 g	31%
ORAC Value: 5,347	Sugars: 7.0 g	

How to Choose

Look for plump, mold-free berries that are uniformly deep black. Keep them in the refrigerator to prolong their life, but check for any moldy berries and remove them before storage.

Strawberry

Strawberries are the world's most popular berries (though technically they aren't berries). There are hundreds of varieties, all with sweet red flesh and yellow seeds on the surface of the fruit. Not only are strawberries delicious, but they have many health benefits. The phenols and anthocyanins in strawberries, as in other berries, are believed to have heart-protecting, cancer-fighting, and anti-inflammatory benefits. Since strawberries are very perishable, it's best not to wash them until right before eating and to wait to remove the caps and stems until after you have washed them. That prevents them from absorbing extra water, which can diminish the texture and flavor.

Nutrition

Strawberries contain high amounts of vitamin C with very little fat and are only 49 calories per cup:

NUTRIENT	AMOUNT	% DAILY VALUE
Vitamin C	89 mg	148%
Calcium	24 mg	2%
Magnesium	20 mg	5%
Potassium	233 mg	7%
Folate	36 mcg	9%
ORAC Value: 3,577	Sugars: 7.4 g	

How to Choose

Conventionally grown strawberries tend to be high in pesticide residue, so it's best to buy organic. Since strawberries do not ripen after they've been picked, choose the reddest ones for the greatest flavor and nutritional benefits. They should be free of mold—sometimes moldy ones are hidden at the bottom of the container, so check carefully. Medium-sized berries, rather than extra large, are usually the most flavorful.

Fruits Low to Medium in Sugar

Papaya

Christopher Columbus called papaya the "fruit of the angels." Apparently, in the New World he noticed that natives ate papayas after large meals and didn't develop any digestive problems. This is because the papain in papaya helps to relieve digestion. A papaya is shaped like a long melon and can be as long as 20 inches, though 7 inches is more typical. The fruit has rich, orange flesh and a core of round, black seeds. Edible, with a peppery flavor, the seeds are anthelmintic, which means they help to expel any worms that may be in the body. The seeds can be mixed with honey and consumed after a main meal or three times a day. Papayas are also rich sources of vitamin C, the B vitamins, folate, potassium, magnesium, and fiber. These nutrients promote the health of the cardiovascular system and help provide protection against colon cancer. Papaya juice also helps to relieve infection in the colon. You can eat a papaya just like a melon, scooping out the flesh with a spoon.

Nutrition

Papaya contains an awesome amount of vitamin C and has just 62 calories in 1 cup:

NUTRIENT	AMOUNT	% DAILY VALUE
Fat	0.38 g	--
Vitamin C	88 mg	146%
Folate	54 mcg	14%
Lycopene	2,651 mcg	--
Beta-Carotene	397 mcg	--
Fiber	2.5 g	10%
ORAC Value: 500 Sugars: 7.8 g		

How to Choose

Papayas should be eaten within a day of purchase. Pick ones that are slightly soft to the touch and have a reddish-orange skin. Fruit with areas of yellow on the skin will take a couple more days to ripen. Hard or totally green papayas should be used only for cooking or in a dish calling for unripe fruit, such as a green papaya salad, popular in Thailand. Be sure to avoid papayas that are really soft. Also avoid bruised skin, though a few black spots on the surface are usually fine.

Grapefruit

Eating a grapefruit is a great way to start the day or makes a refreshing snack. Full of vitamins and minerals, grapefruit is also low in sodium and high in fat-burning enzymes, making it a great choice for weight loss. Eat the white part separating the segments (the pith) in a grapefruit half and you'll get six grams of fiber, a quarter of the recommended daily amount. Even without the pith, you'll still get two grams of fiber. Pectin (a form of soluble fiber) in grapefruit helps to lower blood cholesterol. The lycopene in red-fleshed grapefruits and some other phytonutrients in both red and white grapefruits are thought to inhibit tumor formation.

Nutrition

Just half a medium grapefruit is high in vitamins C and A and low in calories:

NUTRIENT	AMOUNT	% DAILY VALUE
Fat	0.13 g	--
Vitamin C	44 mg	73%
Calcium	15 mg	1.5%
Potassium	178 mg	5%
Beta-carotene	707 mcg	--
Vitamin A	1187 IU	24%

Lycopene	1,453 mcg	--
Folate	13 mcg	3%
Fiber	1.4 g	6%
ORAC Value: 1,548	Sugars: 9.0 g	

How to Choose

Look for grapefruits that are firm, yet slightly soft to the touch, and have a sweet, subtle aroma. Choose fruits that are heavy for their size—they'll be juicy. Imperfections on the skin do not affect the taste or quality of a grapefruit.

Orange

Just one orange supplies more than one and a half times the daily requirement of antioxidant-rich vitamin C. Studies have shown that citrus fruits are particularly powerful in lowering the risk of cancer. The potassium in oranges helps to reduce blood pressure and is believed to protect against stroke. Oranges have incredible health benefits—easy to understand considering that they contain around 170 phytonutrients and 60 flavonoids.

Nutrition

At only 86 calories, one large orange contains amazing amounts of vitamin C and potassium:

NUTRIENT	AMOUNT	% DAILY VALUE
Fat	0.22 g	--
Calcium	74 mg	7%
Potassium	333 mg	10%
Vitamin C	98 mg	163%
Beta-carotene	131 mcg	--
Lutein	238 mcg	--
Fiber	4.4 g	18%
ORAC Value: 1,819	Sugars: 9.0 g	

How to Choose

Buying organic is best since oranges are among the top 20 fruits and vegetables in which pesticide residue is found. Smaller oranges with a thinner rind are usually juicier than very large, thick-skinned fruit. Avoid oranges with any mold or soft spots. Don't go by color: oranges that are slightly green can be just as flavorful and juicy as those with a fully developed orange color.

Pear

If you drink the Detox Blast Smoothie at least weekly, you'll get the amazing health benefits of pears. Pears come in a variety of colors such as yellow, green, brown, red, or a combination of colors. The fruit is full of antioxidants, including copper, which helps protect cells from free radicals. The vitamin C in pears helps cells to fight off infection.

Nutrition

One medium-sized pear is rich in fiber and vitamin C:

NUTRIENT	AMOUNT	% DAILY VALUE
Fat	0.2 g	--
Calcium	16 mg	2%
Magnesium	12 mg	3%
Potassium	212 mg	6%
Vitamin C	7.5 mg	13%
Fiber	5.5 g	22%
ORAC Value: 2,941	Sugars: 9.0 g	

How to Choose

Look for pears that are firm, yet yield slightly to the touch, with no bruises, punctures, or soft spots. It's best to let the fruit ripen at room temperature. Once ripe they are very perishable, so be sure to eat them right away.

Peach

Peaches are among the sweetest and most delicious and nutritious of all fruits. With lots of fiber and more than 80 percent water content, they promote healthy bowel movements, are good for anyone wanting to lose weight, and can even improve the complexion. They're packed with vitamins and minerals that are believed to help prevent cancer. About two peaches provides the daily requirement of vitamin C. Don't peel a peach—eat the flesh and skin to receive the maximum nutrition. Let refrigerated peaches acclimate to room temperature before eating them, as doing so will increase the flavor significantly.

Nutrition

A medium-sized peach provides a powerful amount of potassium at only 58 calories:

NUTRIENT	AMOUNT	% DAILY VALUE
Fat	0.38 g	--
Potassium	285 mg	8%
Vitamin C	9.9 mg	17%
Vitamin A	489 IU	10%
ORAC Value: 1,814	Sugars: 12.4 g	

How to Choose

Because peaches are near the top of the list of fruits and vegetables containing pesticide residue, it's best to buy organic. Choose fruit that is firm to the touch, yet yields slightly to pressure (especially near the stem end), is free of bruises, and has a sweet fragrance. Ripe peaches are highly perishable, so they should be consumed within a couple of days after purchase. Unripe peaches can be ripened in a paper bag punched with holes.

Cantaloupe

This juicy, refreshing round melon with orange flesh and ribbed skin belongs to the same family as the gourd, pumpkin, squash, and cucumber. It is high in beta-carotene, which is converted into vitamin A in the body. This makes cantaloupe one of the best fruit sources of vitamin A and beta-carotene, both needed for vision health. Beta-carotene is also being studied for its potential to reduce the risk of cancer. Cantaloupe is an excellent source of vitamin C as well.

Nutrition

Canteloupes are very high in vitamins A and C, and contain only 54 calories in 1 cup:

NUTRIENT	AMOUNT	% DAILY VALUE
Fat	0.3 g	--
Calcium	14 mg	1.4%
Magnesium	19 mg	5%
Potassium	427 mg	12%
Vitamin C	59 mg	98%
Beta-carotene	3,232 mcg	--
Vitamin A	5,411 IU	108%
Lutein	42 mcg	--
Vitamin K	4 mcg	5%
Fiber	1.4 g	6%
ORAC Value: 315	Sugars: 12.5 g	

How to Choose

Choose a melon that is heavy for its size and has no bruises or overly soft spots. Make sure the rind, underneath the netting of the cantaloupe, has turned yellow or cream. The area where the stem was attached should be free from any remnants of the stem. Smell the cantaloupe to make sure it has a subtly sweet aroma; a strong smell often indicates overripeness. You should hear a hollow sound when you tap a ripe melon with the palm of your hand.

Banana

Bananas are packed with potassium, which helps to lower blood pressure and prevent strokes. The fruit is also effective in protecting against stomach ulcers, improving elimination, and building strong bones. Studies have shown consumption of fruits, especially bananas, may reduce the risk of kidney cancer. The reason is that bananas contain an exceptionally high amount of antioxidant phenols. For the most antioxidants, it's best to eat bananas when they're fully ripe. You'll get a healthy serving of bananas just by drinking the Green Protein Smoothie a couple of times a week. To save time, cut up bananas in advance and store them in containers, two bananas per container, in the freezer and add the frozen bananas to the blender.

Nutrition

Packed with potassium and fiber, one medium-sized banana is just 105 calories:

NUTRIENT	AMOUNT	% DAILY VALUE
Fat	0.39 g	--
Magnesium	32 mg	8%
Potassium	422 mg	12%
Vitamin C	10.3 mg	17%
Beta-carotene	31 mcg	--
Vitamin A	76 IU	2%
Fiber	3.1 g	12%
ORAC Value: 879	Sugars: 14.5 g	

How to Choose

Bananas ripen quickly at room temperature and can be bought when they are still somewhat green. Look for fruit with no bruises or other injuries.

Blueberry

Delectable, with a taste ranging from sweet to tangy, blueberries are fun to pop in your mouth as a snack or toss on your favorite cereal or yogurt. They are also incredibly nutritious. Packed with antioxidants, vitamins, and minerals, they are believed to have amazing health benefits, including boosting the immune system, preventing various forms of cancer, and lowering cholesterol.

Nutrition

Blueberries are packed with vitamins and minerals, while containing very little fat and only 84 calories per cup:

NUTRIENT	AMOUNT	% DAILY VALUE
Fat	0.49 g	--
Calcium	9 mg	15%
Manganese	0.5 mg	25%
Vitamin C	14 mg	24%
Potassium	114 mg	3%
Beta-carotene	47 mcg	--
Fiber	3.6 g	14%
ORAC Value: 6,552	Sugars: 14.8 g	

How to Choose

It's best to buy organic blueberries, since conventionally grown ones are often high in pesticide residue. Blueberries don't ripen after they're picked, so look for plump fruit with a waxy sheen.

The berries should be uniformly blue. Pass up any cartons that have red or purple berries mixed in with the blue, or any cartons that are stained on the bottom. Blueberries last for a couple of weeks if refrigerated, but they should be kept dry, so don't wash the berries until you're ready to eat them.

Dates

These incredibly nourishing little nuggets are an excellent substitute for calorie-laden sweets with added sugar. Rich in vitamins and minerals and a good source of dietary fiber, dates have been shown to be effective in helping prevent anemia, low blood pressure, stomach ulcers, colitis, sexual impotency, and nervous conditions.

Nutrition

At 66 calories each, a date may be high in calories and sugars, but it is a good source of fiber:

NUTRIENT	AMOUNT	% DAILY VALUE
Fat	0.04 g	--
Calcium	15 mg	1.5%
Potassium	167 mg	5%
Beta-carotene	21 mcg	--
Fiber	2 g	8%
ORAC Value: 2,387	Sugars: 15.6 g	

How to Choose

When choosing dates, look for ones that are pitted and plump and look shiny rather than dry. California dates are the most commonly available variety; whole (with pits) are usually freshest and moistest, but are not as convenient for cooking. You can select California dates from the bulk section at most natural grocery stores. Prepackaged California dates are also good, but double check to make sure they look fresh. The exceptionally large, sweet, and meaty Medjool dates are also an excellent option; they are widely available at many grocery stores.

Pineapple

It's easy to understand why the pineapple is second to the banana as America's favorite tropical fruit. With a delicious balance of tartness and sweetness, pineapple is refreshing and juicy. It is packed with vitamin C, which helps to prevent or reduce the severity of arthritis, heart disease, and asthma and may be significant in reducing the risk of cancer. Pineapple is also an excellent source of the trace mineral manganese, which works with enzymes in the body to disarm free radicals.

Nutrition

Pineapple has large amounts of magnesium and vitamin C, while containing only 82 calories per cup:

NUTRIENT	AMOUNT	% DAILY VALUE
Fat	0.2 g	--
Calcium	21 mg	2%
Magnesium	20 mg	5%
Potassium	180 mg	5%
Manganese	1.5 mg	75%
ORAC Value: 884	Sugars: 16.3 g	

How to Choose

A ripe pineapple should be heavy for its size. While larger pineapples have more edible flesh, there is usually no difference in flavor between bigger and smaller pineapples. A pineapple stops ripening once it is picked, so look for one that is more golden yellow than green. It should also be free of dark spots, bruises, or darkened eyes. A good pineapple will have a sweet, fragrant smell at the stem end. Avoid any pineapples that smell musty, fermented, or sour.

Apple

Nutritious, delicious apples are filled with vitamins and minerals as well fiber to keep you feeling satisfied and full. Apples develop acids that stimulate the flow of saliva and encourage digestion. They contain antioxidants, cancer-fighting flavonoids and pectin, which is believed to lower cholesterol and high blood pressure. If that weren't enough, they also help remove plaque from teeth. Eat an apple with the skin on to be sure you receive the maximum nutritional benefits.

Nutrition

Apples are high in vitamin C and fiber, while providing very little fat and only 95 calories for a medium-sized fruit:

NUTRIENT	AMOUNT	% DAILY VALUE
Fat	0.3 g	--
Vitamin C	8.4 mg	14%
Vitamin A	98 IU	2%
Magnesium	9 mg	2%
Potassium	195 mg	6%
Vitamin K	4 mcg	5%
Fiber	4.4 g	18%
ORAC Value: 3,082	Sugars: 18.9 g	

How to Choose

Conventionally grown apples are among the fruits that tend to contain pesticide residue, so it's best to buy organic. Look for brightly colored, firm fruit with a smooth skin. Storing apples in the refrigerator will increase their shelf life; some apples can be stored for up to two months refrigerated.

Cherries

Cherries are a wonderful and nutritious treat. They are packed with antioxidants that fight free radicals and are believed to help prevent cancer and heart disease, as well as to slow the aging process. A diet that includes cherries has been known to decrease body fat, cholesterol, and inflammation. Cherries also contain melatonin, which helps to regulate sleep patterns.

Nutrition

Cherries have a high amount of potassium and vitamin C, with only 97 calories per cup:

NUTRIENT	AMOUNT	% DAILY VALUE
Fat	0.31 g	--
Calcium	20 mg	2%
Magnesium	17 mg	4%
Phosphorus	32 mg	3%
Potassium	342 mg	10%
Vitamin C	10.8 mg	18%
Fiber	3.2 g	13%
ORAC Value: 3,365	Sugars: 19.74 g	

How to Choose

The darker the cherries, the sweeter they will taste. Look for cherries that are free of bruises and mold and are slightly firm to the touch. And, of course, make sure they are nice and plump.

Mango

Sometimes referred to as the king of fruit, mangoes offer incredible nutritional benefits. In many parts of the world they're a household remedy and are believed to be particularly helpful in treating inflammation and other conditions of the kidneys as well as in reducing fevers and combating acidity and poor digestion. The fruit is a good source of antioxidants and vitamin C, which help in preventing many cancers, and fiber, which reduces the risk of colon cancer. To get rid of clogged skin pores, simply remove the pulp from a mango and apply it to the skin for ten minutes before washing.

Nutrition

Mangoes have a fantastic amount of vitamin C in just 1 cup:

NUTRIENT	AMOUNT	% DAILY VALUE
Fat	0.63 g	--
Calcium	18 mg	2%
Magnesium	16 mg	4%
Potassium	277 mg	8%
Vitamin C	60 mg	100%
Choline	12.5 mg	--
Vitamin A	1,785 IU	36%
Fiber	2.6 g	10%
ORAC Value: 1,002	Sugars: 22.5 g	

How to Choose

To find a good mango, pick one that's plump and heavy for its size. Avoid any mangoes that are mushy or have brown marks. Color by itself is not the best indication of ripeness—mangoes come in shades of green, yellow, and red, and many show more than one color. A gentle squeeze is a better test of ripeness. A ripe mango will be slightly soft and will have a sweet, fruity aroma at the stem end. Unripe fruit will ripen in a few days at room temperature.

12

The Dirty Dozen and Buying Organic

Never believe that a few caring people can't change the world. For, indeed, that's all who ever have.

—Margaret Mead

How important is it to buy organic when eating a diet rich in fruits and vegetables? Very...depending on what you are eating.

Chances are you've heard of the Dirty Dozen. These are the 12 most important fruits and vegetables when it comes to buying organic, as they are the most susceptible to absorbing pesticides and transferring the ill effects of industrial farming to consumers. For example, peaches, the fruit nearest the top of the list, tested for 67 chemicals.

The list changes somewhat from year to year but usually includes thin-skinned fruits such as apples, blueberries, strawberries, and tomatoes. The Environmental Working Group (www.ewg.org) puts together the Dirty Dozen list each year. To find the most up-to-date list you can simply do an Internet search for "dirty dozen" and the current year. In 2011, the Dirty Dozen was:

1. Apples
2. Celery
3. Strawberries
4. Peaches
5. Spinach
6. Nectarines (imported)
7. Grapes (imported)
8. Sweet bell peppers
9. Potatoes
10. Blueberries (domestic)
11. Lettuce
12. Kale/collard greens

While it's a good idea to pay attention to the Dirty Dozen list this year, you should also abide by these simple rules: if you eat the skin, go organic. Even when you don't eat the skin, if it's a fleshy fruit with thin skin, go organic. The same rules apply to vegetables, with the added caveat to always go organic with leafy greens like lettuce and spinach.

Thanks to their thick skins (not normally consumed), the following fruits and vegetables are considered safe to consume, even when raised through questionable farming practices. While it's still a good idea to buy organic whenever possible, you can enjoy these Clean 15 at any time as they have little to no trace of pesticides:

1. Onions
2. Sweet corn
3. Pineapples
4. Avocados
5. Asparagus
6. Sweet peas
7. Mangoes
8. Eggplants
9. Cantaloupe (domestic)
10. Kiwi
11. Cabbage
12. Watermelon
13. Sweet potatoes
14. Grapefruit
15. Mushrooms

If organic produce isn't readily available in your area, sticking to the Clean 15 will reduce your pesticide exposure by about 90 percent.

Until you are able to completely change to an organic diet, start with organic versions of the produce on the Dirty Dozen list. If cost is a concern, a great way to buy organic at reasonable prices is to join a food cooperative if one is available in your area.

The Scary World of Food Production

Did you know that while the muscle of conventionally farmed animals is usually clean, the fat is often contaminated with hormones and antibiotics?

So, it's a good idea to go organic when you're choosing meat, dairy, eggs, and even fish, to avoid pesticides, fertilizers, and other toxins. Even if cows, pigs, and chickens aren't injected with hormones and antibiotics, they most likely are fed corn that's been grown with chemical fertilizers, because 90 percent of all soybeans and 60 percent of all corn grown conventionally in the U.S. are genetically modified.

The best way to avoid ingesting chemicals and other toxins is to eliminate dairy, eggs, and meats from your diet or to choose organically produced versions.

Another Reason to Go Organic: Save the Planet

We live in a time when we have the opportunity to change our behavior and quite literally make the world a better place. To actually know we have that opportunity is the ultimate gift of realization. All of us can be proactive and know that we have the power to make a difference. That potential for positive change lies within each of us. By making better choices and living with increasing awareness, you positively affect everything around you. The changes you make can seem simple yet be profound.

When you eat organic, which is more affordable than you might think, you contribute to your own health as well as to a healthier planet by supporting farmers who care for the land with positive farming practices. An increase in demand for nutritious, organically produced foods will spur those who are not farming in a sustainable way to change for the better. Each one of us can significantly reduce the amount of waste and toxins we contribute to the planet, whether that's with the foods we choose to eat or with anything else in our lives.

A friend of mine told me that when he orders takeout from his favorite local restaurants, he brings his own to-go container with him instead of having the restaurant use disposable materials. I hadn't thought about that before, but what a concept. If you have a favorite restaurant you order from, I'm sure they would be happy to accommodate you to help reduce your own waste and theirs.

It's incredible what can happen when we all work together. *Can you imagine the difference it would make if each one of us brought a reusable container each time we ordered takeout?* It seems to me we are finally beginning to realize the power of positive change, which is possible when we choose to work together in small and great ways. The reality is that we are all one. If we want to have a healthy planet and healthy homes, it's up to all of us to contribute to that in any way we can.

Recently I ate a conventionally grown apple (one of the Dirty Dozen), and even after I washed it, I could taste the pesticides. After consuming that apple, I decided I would eat only organic apples from that point forward. We can make better choices. While it might take a little longer to change the air we breathe, we can at least make an empowered choice by changing the food we eat. By doing this, we will see the world around us transform in a positive way.

You've probably noticed that grocery stores are carrying more and more organic and natural foods. Not long ago, when I was in a large chain store, I began talking to one of the managers. He pointed to an aisle with sugar-laden cereals and said he believed that in time more and more of the processed foods would go away and we would increasingly see organic and natural foods filling the shelves at affordable prices. Hallelujah.

The bottom line is, we are where we are, so what are we going to do now with the tools, knowledge, and wisdom we have? Instead of lamenting, do something. Make some small or significant change for the better. You might not think your actions are affecting anything around you, but they are and they will. In addition to making better choices, together we can hope that in time we will evolve to an increasingly conscious, positive, and beneficial way of caring for ourselves, each other, and the earth.

PART III

Life After the Fresh Fruit Cleanse

13

After the Fresh Fruit Cleanse

Foods contain nutrients for normal metabolic function, and when problems arise, they result from imbalances in nutrient intake and from harmful interactions with other factors. For the two out of three adult Americans who do not smoke and do not drink excessively, one personal choice seems to influence long-term health prospects more than any other—what we eat.

—C. Everett Koop, M.D., Surgeon General, 1981–1989

When you finish the Fresh Fruit Cleanse, you should feel good about yourself. You accomplished your goal, progressing farther along the path to health and well-being, but, now is not the time to be complacent. It's important to keep your focus on your larger vision in life, whether it's to steadily improve your health, lose weight, or detoxify your body for a new start. Here's information you need to adapt to life after the Fresh Fruit Cleanse and how to prepare for the next cleanse, while holding onto everything you learned about yourself during the cleanse you just completed.

10 Tips for Ending the Cleanse

1. Eat healthy foods, choosing organic as much as possible.
2. Continue to enjoy the recipes in this book, and find other healthy recipes you like.
3. Exercise. Practice yoga and meditation.
4. Stay on the path of health and well-being, and let go of any addictions, such as coffee, alcohol, or nicotine.
5. Surround yourself with positive people who are inspired to be healthy, too.
6. Set an example for others by embodying health and well-being, but don't try to convert others to your transformed lifestyle.
7. Live your life to the fullest and know that as you grow well, everything in your life will grow well, too.
8. Laugh often, forgive quickly, and love deeply. Life is too short for drama and pettiness. Be grateful, love your Higher Power, and love your neighbor as yourself.
9. Envision and plan your next cleanse.
10. Believe in yourself always and never give up.

Foods to Moderate

During the Fresh Fruit Cleanse you eliminated alcohol, caffeine, refined sugar, processed foods, gluten, flour, eggs, meat, dairy, soy, corn, and potatoes. *So, what kind of positive, health-conscious choices will you make now that you've completed the Fresh Fruit Cleanse?* While that's entirely up to you, it's important to realize that certain foods, including many you eliminated during the cleanse, can cause allergic reactions and have negative physical effects on your body. In the United States today, eight of the top ten causes of diseases are directly related to diet. To feel your best, a primarily vegan lifestyle is the healthiest diet you can follow. A diet rich in fresh fruits and vegetables, and packed full of vitamins and minerals, is optimal for a healthy body, mind, and spirit.

If you plan on eating any of the following foods after you finish the Fresh Fruit Cleanse, it's important to consciously reintroduce them, one at a time, back into your diet to fully experience how each food makes you feel. This way, you will notice any adverse or unhealthy side effects, such as toxicity, lethargy, or bloating.

Alcohol
Caffeine
Corn
Dairy
Eggs
Fish
Flour
Gluten
Meat
Refined sugar
Soy

You may find that you now have no desire, or perhaps much less desire, for any or all of these foods or for caffeine or alcohol. I've found the less I consume these items, the healthier I feel. The Fresh Fruit Cleanse encourages moderation in all choices in life. It's fine to have a cup of coffee, a special dessert, or a glass of wine occasionally, but many of the items in the list are the biggest sources of food allergies and intolerances and the greatest causes of weight gain, high levels of acidity, toxicity, and disease in the body.

Let go of the idea that a particular food is bad. What's most important is how it makes you feel. *How do you know if you have an allergy or intolerance to certain foods, and what are the symptoms?* For starters, it's important to understand the difference between food allergies and food intolerances. Also keep in mind that, if you think you have symptoms, a health care professional can determine whether you have a food allergy or a food intolerance and can help you develop the best nutritional plan for your health and well-being.

Food Allergies

The most common food allergies are to peanuts, tree nuts (pecans, walnuts, and almonds), fish, shellfish, milk, eggs, wheat, and soy. A food allergy is an immune system response. When the body mistakes a food as harmful (the culprit is usually a protein in the food), it creates antibodies in the immune system to fight it.

Some of the most common food allergy symptoms are nausea, diarrhea, stomach pain, a rash or hives, chest pain, swelling of the airways to the lungs, shortness of breath, and itchy skin.

Food allergies are often hereditary. If you have any of the above symptoms, you may have a food allergy. This is why it's important to slowly reintroduce any foods or substances back into your diet after the Fresh Fruit Cleanse, so you can be as aware as possible of the effect they have on your body. Food allergies affect about 2 to 4 percent of adults and 6 to 8 percent of children. The usual way to treat a food allergy is to avoid the food completely. If it turns out you are allergic to wheat or another hard-to-avoid item, a dietitian or nutritionist can help you find healthy alternatives.

Food Intolerances

Unlike a food allergy, a food intolerance is a digestive response rather than an immune system response. Food intolerances occur when something in a food irritates the digestive system or when the body is unable to properly break down or digest a food. The most common food intolerance is to lactose, found in milk and other dairy products, affecting about 10 percent of Americans.

Some of the most common food intolerance symptoms are nausea, diarrhea, stomach pain, vomiting, heartburn, and gas, cramps, or bloating, as well as headache and irritability.

Food intolerances result because a person lacks the necessary enzymes to digest certain foods properly, and they are often dose related. This means that certain foods can be OK in small quantities, but they can have adverse side effects when consumed in larger amounts. Someone who is lactose intolerant may be able to eat one piece of cheese or drink a single glass of milk but could become sick when consuming larger quantities of dairy in a single sitting.

Reintroducing Foods into Your Diet

It's often difficult to know whether you have a food allergy caused by a certain food if you eliminate it for only a short period. To really know if you are allergic, eliminate that food for an entire month. This is called an elimination diet. Because the Fresh Fruit Cleanse is both a detoxification and elimination program, your senses about certain foods will be heightened after you complete the cleanse. You may find you are immediately aware of which foods make you feel your best and which foods don't. Slowly reintroduce the items on the list of foods to moderate—perhaps one item every three days—and notice how you feel. Does that food make you feel positive, energized, healthy, alive, and light or does it make you feel heavy, fatigued, tired, and depressed? Once you become aware of the effect of certain foods on your body, you'll know what to eat simply by asking yourself this question: *How will this food make me feel?*

When to Eat Fruit

There are many different beliefs about when it's best to eat fruit, but the general rule of thumb is to eat it on an empty stomach. The reason is that your body will absorb the maximum nutritional benefit of the fruit without having to digest it with any other food at the same time. Fruit and fruit juice are the most easily digested foods you can eat. The vitamins and minerals are digested and absorbed into the bloodstream in about a half hour, and the glucose is utilized by the brain.

When you eat fruit, it's best to wait about 30 minutes before eating any other food. Also, after eating a meal, it's ideal to wait two hours before consuming any fruit. This will keep the food from putrefying and fermenting in the stomach, which can happen when fruit is digested at the same time as other food. Some cultures eat fruit as dessert, but this is actually wasting many of its nutritional benefits. To get the most out of fruit and to feel your best, eat fruit by itself. When you do this, you just might find you don't need as much other food and that you feel full, healthy, and satisfied on mostly fruit alone.

Healthy Dairy Alternatives

If you are going to eat dairy, choose organic products. But if you're willing to eliminate dairy, you'll be happy to learn that there are many wonderful dairy alternatives. Why do I recommend eating less dairy and opting for alternatives? Cow's milk, cheese, butter, cream, yogurt, cottage cheese, ghee, kefir, and whey are all incredibly mucus-forming foods. Goat's milk is much less mucus forming than cow's milk, though it's still best to enjoy goat's milk in moderation.

Although mucus is necessary to keep interior linings of the body moist, dairy foods can cause the body to produce cloudy, thick, sticky mucus, which is unhealthy for the digestive and intestinal tract and the rest of the body. Dairy products are also very acid forming—and a high level of acidity in the body is believed to be the cause of many diseases.

Here are my favorite dairy alternatives:

Milk

- Organic vanilla almond milk
- Organic vanilla rice milk

Yogurt

- So Delicious coconut milk yogurt (any flavor)

Cheese

- Daiya dairy-free cheese

Ice Cream

- Coconut Bliss coconut milk ice cream (any flavor)
- So Delicious coconut milk ice cream (any flavor)

It's possible to find almond milk and rice milk at almost any grocery store these days. Coconut milk yogurt is also becoming widely available. Daiya dairy-free cheese is still mostly available at natural health food stores such as Whole Foods or Sprouts, but I hope it will be at more grocery stores soon.

Gluten vs. Gluten-Free

The gluten-free industry has been growing because about 0.5 percent of the population is intolerant to gluten, or the protein component found in wheat, barley, and rye. These proteins, known as peptides, are called gliadin (in wheat), secalin (in rye), and hordein (in barley). Gluten is the second most common food intolerance in the country. Some people must avoid gluten completely because of celiac disease, a hypersensitivity to the peptides affecting the small intestine and the body's ability to absorb nutrients from food. Symptoms of celiac disease include diarrhea, abdominal pain, and bloating. Gluten allergies are also common and must be treated seriously; professional medical attention is recommended.

Many people believe that eating less gluten will keep them from gaining weight, but this is simply not true. It's not the gluten that causes weight gain, but the sugar added to many wheat and flour products. Although there are many wonderful gluten-free alternatives, most of the products are made from highly refined carbohydrates and are therefore low in fiber and B vitamins. However, some gluten-free products are made with nuts, seeds, and other healthy ingredients. Mary's Gone Crackers, for example, are made from brown rice, quinoa, flax seeds, and sesame seeds—all organic. The original flavor is one of my favorite crackers to top with hummus.

If you don't have an allergy to gluten but prefer to eat gluten-free products, make sure your diet is well rounded and nutritious. Eat nuts, which are full of protein, fiber, and vitamin E, and, use nut-based flours when baking. Also, it's important to eat beans, also packed with fiber and protein, as well as brown rice and whole grains like quinoa, buckwheat, and amaranth. Rice and grains make excellent side dishes instead of pastas or breads. Tapioca flour can be substituted for wheat flour in many recipes to make the recipe gluten-free. It's best to combine tapioca flour with other gluten-free flours like potato starch and white rice. To make a good quantity of a gluten-free flour blend, mix 6 cups white rice flour, 2 cups potato starch flour, and 1 cup tapioca flour. Arrowroot, amaranth, quinoa, millet, and buckwheat are also great substitutes for wheat.

Here are a few of my favorite gluten-free alternatives:

Crackers

- Mary's Gone Crackers
- Blue Diamond Nut-Thins

Pasta

- Ancient Harvest Quinoa pasta
- Tinkyada Pasta Joy Ready Organic Brown Rice Pasta Spirals
- Spaghetti squash

To Soy or Not to Soy

Many people who are vegetarians turn to soy as a healthy meat or dairy substitute, but the truth is that soy may not be the ideal food for you. While soy is high in protein, over 90 percent of soy products are genetically modified, and soy is one of the most pesticide-contaminated foods. As in anything else, moderation is key; a little tofu here or there is OK, but don't make a habit of eating heavily processed or manufactured soy foods. Other than edamame, all soy products are processed. If you are going to eat soy, choose organic products. It's best to eat a wide variety of foods that are as close to the earth as possible and require the least amount of processing. There are other, more natural ways to increase the amount of protein in your diet.

Healthy Plant Proteins

We all know that protein is essential for good health. Over time, with cleansing and healthy living practices, it's natural to gravitate toward a more plant-based diet. *So, how do you make sure you'll get enough protein when you are eating a diet rich in whole grains, vegetables, and fruits?*

Dairy products and meats are mucus-forming foods and can cause the body to feel heavy and lethargic. Even so, you may think that you need dairy and meat to supply your body with protein, but the truth is that plant-based foods are packed with protein, especially spirulina, garlic, seeds, and nuts. One of the biggest misconceptions is that a vegetarian or mostly plant-based diet won't give your body enough protein. This just isn't true. In order to be optimally healthy, only 10 percent of calories consumed need to be protein, and it's better if that protein comes from plants rather than animals. In fact, too much animal protein is believed to be linked to kidney stones as well as liver and colon cancer.

Fruits

Apples
Bananas
Cantaloupes
Grapefruits
Grapes
Honeydew melons
Mandarin oranges
Oranges
Papayas
Peaches
Pears
Pineapples
Strawberries
Watermelons

Vegetables

Artichokes
Beets
Broccoli
Brussels sprouts
Cabbages
Cauliflower
Cucumbers
Eggplants
Green peas
Green peppers
Lettuces
Kale
Mustard greens
Mushrooms
Onions
Potatoes
Spinach
Tomatoes
Watercress
Zucchinis

Legumes

- Garbanzo beans
- Kidney beans
- Lentils
- Lima beans
- Navy beans
- Soy beans
- Split peas

Grains

- Barley
- Brown rice
- Buckwheat
- Millet
- Oatmeal
- Quinoa
- Rye
- Wheat
- Wheat germ
- Wild rice

Nuts and Seeds

- Almonds
- Cashews
- Hazelnuts
- Hemp seeds
- Peanuts
- Pumpkin seeds
- Sunflower seeds
- Walnuts

Fats

Fat is the most concentrated energy source available to the body. In recent years there's been a lot of talk about the different kinds of fats. Read food labels, and stay away from trans fats or partially hydrogenated fats; they are synthetically processed fats that have hydrogen added to them (hydrogenation) to prolong their shelf life. Even consuming as little as three or four grams per day of these fats can harm the body, contributing to heart disease, high blood pressure, diabetes, and cancer. Other types of fats include saturated fats, known as "bad" fats, and healthy fats like omega-3 fatty acids.

Saturated Fats

We've all heard about these fats, which are found mainly in meats and dairy products and also in fatty foods like chips and pastries. What makes saturated fats bad for you is overconsumption—when you consume more than the recommended daily allowance of them—or when the fats have been damaged by heat, oxygen, or unnatural farming practices. Damaged fats can lead to a buildup of plaque that impairs blood circulation. Examples of damaged fats include:

- Dairy products, including cheese and ice cream made from pasteurized milk
- Powdered milk
- Powdered eggs
- Meats cooked at high temperatures, especially when fried or deep fried
- Any vegetable oils with the words "shortening," "partially hydrogenated vegetable oil," or "hydrogenated vegetable oil" on the label
- All hydrogenated oils, including margarine

Saturated fats, damaged or not, can raise LDL blood cholesterol (the bad cholesterol) levels, clogging arteries and veins. They are also believed to cause certain types of cancers. Most experts recommend that the daily intake of saturated fats be kept below 10 percent of your total daily caloric intake.

Unsaturated Fats

Unsaturated fats, including omega-3 and omega-6 essential fatty acids (EFAs), are the healthy fats known to lower cholesterol and improve good cholesterol (HDL). They are essential to good health.

The ideal amount of EFAs is 10 to 20 percent of your total caloric intake, and the suggested dietary ratio of omega-6 to omega-3 fatty acids is 2:1–4:1. Because of the proliferation of vegetable oils, margarines, processed foods, and convenience foods, all of which contain high levels of omega-6s and virtually no omega-3s, that ratio is approaching an unhealthy 30:1. The best sources of omega-6s and omega-3s are flax seeds and hemp seeds and their oils. Drinking the Green Protein Smoothie or the Detox Blast Smoothie, or adding flax or hemp seeds or their oils to any of your favorite smoothies, will supply your body with the healthiest and most nutritious fats. All oils made from organic seeds provide a perfect balance of omega-6s and omega-3s. Mixing your favorite seed-based oil with a touch of balsamic vinegar and dipping a piece of sprouted bread in it is also a great way to get essential fatty acids. The healthiest way to eat flax seeds, for maximum EFA absorption, is raw and freshly ground. Follow this simple recipe for optimal health:

¼ cup whole flax seeds (freshly ground right before use)

1 cup water

Soak the ground flax seeds in the water overnight. Stir in the morning, and drink to your health.

The fats you eat are very important, so let's look at some of the different fats and how they can improve or affect your health.

Omega-3s Studies show that 99 percent of Americans do not consume enough omega-3s. These essential fatty acids containing alpha-linolenic and eicosapentaenoic acid (EPA) are found in flax seeds, hemp seeds, chia seeds, pumpkin seeds, walnuts, soybeans, dark leafy greens (especially kale and collard greens), and cold water fish like salmon, halibut, and tuna, as well as fish oils.

The Best Oils for Cooking

Oils from seeds rich in essential fatty acids, such as flax seed, pumpkin seed, and walnut oils, should never be used for frying or sautéing because they produce toxic substances when heated. They are best used in cold dishes or drizzled over cooked food. Virgin coconut, safflower, avocado, and red palm oils are best for cooking, because a large percentage of saturated fats in them remain stable and undamaged by heat. Many vegetable oils are damaged when heated. That's why you're better off using cold-pressed olive oil raw rather than cooking with it.

Omega-3s are believed to reduce inflammation and the incidence of cancer, heart disease, arthritis, osteoporosis, and depression, and can help assist with weight loss since they come from healthy foods. Found in high concentrations in the brain, omega-3s are vital for memory, performance, and behavioral functions, including alleviating depression. They also improve skin and hair and reduce blood pressure. During pregnancy, it's important to eat healthy amounts of omega-3s to prevent fetuses from developing nerve or vision problems.

Omega-6s Omega-6s, which contain linoleic and gamma-linoleic acids (GLA), are found primarily in raw nuts and seeds, legumes, and unsaturated vegetable oils, such as borage, grape-seed, primrose, sesame, and soybean oils. The linoleic acid is converted into GLA. GLA converts to hormone-like substances that help to block or promote inflammation in the cardiovascular, circulatory, neurological, and gastrointestinal systems. It's best to consume any EFAs in their raw, unheated, whole food state to maximize their health benefits. Heat destroys essential fatty acids. Even worse, it creates harmful free radicals.

Super Foods

These foods found in nature have amazing medicinal and nutritional benefits because of their high level of vitamins, minerals, phytonutrients, and antioxidants. Studies show that super foods like spirulina, maca, raw cacao, hemp seeds, and young coconut are incredible for your health and well-being. The nutritional evidence for them has been solidly proved, although many medical claims have yet to be validated by mainstream medicine. I have experimented with many different super foods and absolutely believe they are healing and medicinal.

When you consider that organic foods have only 20 to 30 percent more nutrients than conventional foods, you can see why it's important to find alternative ways to increase your intake of foods high in vitamins, minerals, and antioxidants. Eating a diet rich in fruits and vegetables is a good first step. And starting a garden is also beneficial, as homegrown produce has 50 percent more nutrients than conventionally farmed produce. Increasing your daily intake of vitamins and minerals through super foods is also important and, quite possibly, essential for your health. You will feel better, healthier, fuller, and more alive with less food, because you are eating food packed with nutrition.

Many people wonder how they can afford to include super foods in their diet. My feeling is that it's essential to incorporate these incredible foods and to find a way to afford them. For example, if you normally go to the movies and eat popcorn or buy a bag of unhealthy chips at the grocery store every week, stop spending your money on food that can't heal you and won't make you feel your best over the long term. Instead, fill up with a Green Protein Smoothie before you go to the movies and forget the popcorn. Or if you're watching a movie at home, pop your own popcorn so it's healthier. If you allow yourself to rearrange your budget to afford super foods, you will notice a difference in how you look and feel in just a few weeks.

Hemp Seeds

The first recorded use of hemp as medicine was around 2300 BC, when the Chinese Emperor Shen-Nung prescribed hemp for the treatment of constipation, gout, malaria, menstrual problems, rheumatism, and beriberi. He classified *chu-ma* (female hemp) as one of the elixirs of immortality.

The omega-3s and omega-6s in hemp seeds are highly beneficial for cellular health and are perfectly balanced to meet human requirements for essential fatty acids. The seeds are an excellent vegan alternative to fish oils because they boost the immune system, improve memory, and help the body to stay warm in cold environments.

Flax Seeds

Flax seeds were used for medicinal and culinary purposes in ancient Greece and Rome. Today we know more about why they're good for us. In addition to being an excellent source of omega-3 fatty acids, flax seeds are full of fiber, which is essential for colon health. Fiber also helps you to feel full and relieves the temptation to eat unhealthy foods.

Flax seed oil does not contain the fiber or phytochemicals found in the seeds, so it's best to eat ground flax seeds to receive the full nutritional benefits. If you purchase flax seed oil or pre-ground flax seeds, make sure they're in an opaque container (exposure to light causes rancidity) and keep the container in your refrigerator. Pre-ground flax seeds can also be stored in the freezer.

Chia Seeds

The Aztecs ate the chia seed to improve their endurance. They called it their "running food" because messengers could run all day on just a handful. The Aztecs used chia as medicine and prized it more highly than gold. It is higher in protein than wheat, corn, rice, oats, barley, amaranth, and soy. It's also packed with antioxidants and is an abundant source of omega-3 fatty acids, which is excellent for cardiovascular and mental health. Chia is the highest known whole-food source of omega-3.

Spirulina

With an ORAC score of 61,900, spirulina is amazing for your health. The chlorophyll in spirulina aids in cleansing and detoxifying the body. Leafy green vegetables are a great source of chlorophyll, but nothing is as rich in chlorophyll as spirulina and chlorella, two blue-green freshwater microalgae. These microalgae also have the highest protein content of any food, making them a complete protein high in essential fatty acids, vitamins, minerals, and glycolipids, which provide energy and serve as markers for cells to communicate with each other. Spirulina has significantly more protein than fish, beef, or tofu, making it an excellent option for vegetarians—or anyone wanting a healthier diet.

Spirulina contains both water- and fat-soluble vitamins and is a rich source of B12, more than double the amount in beef liver. It also contains a spectrum of B vitamins, all of which help to release energy from food and maintain a healthy nervous system, and it contains much more calcium than spinach or milk do.

Research shows that eating a diet rich in beta-carotenes gives the body real anti-cancer protection, and spirulina contains ten times more beta-carotene than carrots. A study done in

Israel showed that natural beta-carotene, like the kind found in spirulina, is far more effective in its anti-cancer properties than synthetically made products.

Spirulina is available in capsules, tablets, and powders and has even been incorporated in foods such as energy bars as well as in smoothies sold at many juice bars. It's generally cultivated in natural or artificial lakes, harvested, and freeze dried.

Maca

According to folklore, Incan warriors used to eat maca before going into battle because they believed it would give them invincible strength and stamina. The reality is it probably did. Also known as Peruvian ginseng, maca grows in the Andes at altitudes of 14,500 feet, where few other plants can survive. It's an energy booster that is believed to relieve stress, insomnia, depression, and PMS, as well as heighten libido, increase testosterone levels, enhance fertility, and improve athletic performance. One of its most powerful qualities is that it's an adaptogen, meaning it helps the body adapt to stress and return to a normal state. Maca has a pleasant malty, butterscotch-like flavor perfect in any smoothie.

Magical Maca Potion

Makes 2 servings

2 cups vanilla almond milk
dash of vanilla extract
1 tablespoon maca powder
pinch of ground cinnamon, to taste
agave nectar or honey, to taste
2 tablespoons coconut oil or butter
⅛–⅓ cup raw cacao (optional)

Combine all ingredients in a blender and blend well. Drink and enjoy.

Raw Cacao

Chocolate in its raw form is said to be one of the most medicinal and healthiest foods on the planet. Regular consumption of raw chocolate is even believed to increase longevity. When the cacao bean is excessively heated, processed, melted, chemicalized, and added to dairy products, it loses its brain nutrition and psychoactive properties. The antioxidants, mood elevation, and aphrodisiac qualities still remain but are diminished by cooking.

Raw chocolate is also one of the most antioxidant-rich foods, outdoing even the acai berry, red wine, and green tea. It offers a healthy dose of minerals, including sulfur, which builds strong nails and hair and promotes beautiful skin by detoxifying the liver and supporting a healthy pancreas.

Coconut Water and Oil

Coconut water is the best natural source of electrolytes as well as an excellent source of potassium, calcium, and magnesium. It also contains small amounts of folate, a B-complex vitamin, along with other micronutrients and phytochemicals, which may explain the feeling of well-being and general health that comes with regularly drinking the water of young coconuts. Coconut water is so good for hydration that it has even been used successfully as a short-term substitute for IV fluid.

I highly recommend coconut oil for cooking. It is antibacterial, antiviral, antiparasitic, and antifungal, making it effective in fighting infections. The oil is also highly alkaline. It purifies the blood, is believed to prevent heart disease, and has been shown to have anti-cancer benefits. It's excellent for diabetics because it supplies energy to the cells without affecting blood sugar or insulin levels.

Honey

Regularly consuming honey, just like eating raw chocolate, is believed to increase longevity. Nutrient-packed honey is a universal medicine and sweetener. It's nature's richest source of healing enzymes. Research indicates that honey improves reflexes, mental alertness, and even IQ. Different honeys may provide additional benefits. Manuka honey from the New Zealand rainforest, for example, is believed to have antifungal, antibiotic, and antiviral qualities.

Eat honey raw. When cooked, it loses its enzymes. You can buy honey from local farmer's markets or from beekeepers who confirm the honey has been heated no higher than 110°F. Raw honey soothes sore throats, helps heal cuts and burns, makes food more digestible, and assists in weight loss by increasing the body's metabolism. So, indulge healthily in honey and enjoy one of the most wonderful and nutritiously medicinal foods in the world.

Garlic

Garlic has been used for over 5,000 years to cure all kinds of physical ailments. It is considered to be a food that promotes optimal health and longevity. Garlic is actually a member of the lily family and a cousin to onions, leeks, chives, and shallots. Garlic is highest in the mineral manganese and provides vitamin B6, vitamin C, and some selenium. Numerous studies show that eating garlic regularly improves blood pressure, triglycerides, and cholesterol levels. It also helps to lessen the "stickiness" of platelets and may inhibit plaque and calcification of arteries. One study of men and women showed those who ate more garlic had a significantly lower risk of certain oral, prostate, and kidney cancers compared to those who ate the least. Garlic may also be helpful in reducing the pain of arthritis because it contains certain compounds that inhibit enzymes that cause inflammation. However, most people don't eat enough garlic to get the nutrients it offers. It takes about four cloves to provide 10 percent of the body's daily value for manganese.

Healing Herbs

Turmeric

A member of the ginger family, turmeric is used worldwide as a culinary seasoning. Curcumin, the active ingredient in turmeric possesses medicinal properties and for thousands of years has been used as a cleansing herb in India and Southeast Asia to treat throat ulcers, inflammation, skin wounds, poor digestion, jaundice, arthritis, and cancer.

Turmeric is also a powerful herb for the liver, rivaling milk thistle in its ability to treat hepatitis and improve liver function. It helps to stimulate the production of bile to break down fats, and it improves peristalsis, the rhythmic contractions that move food through the intestinal tract.

Milk Thistle

This plant, used medicinally since the fourth century BC has antioxidant, anti-inflammatory, antibacterial, and anti-cancer properties. It is considered the remedy of choice for protecting the liver, kidneys, and other capillary-rich tissues. A large number of clinical studies conducted in the past 40 years have shown that milk thistle extract protects and regenerates liver cells. It also helps to reduce blood cholesterol because it decreases the manufacture of liver cholesterol while increasing the secretion of bile and other toxins from the liver. Milk thistle has been known to prevent gallstones and rejuvenate kidney tissue as well. Take 200 to 600 mg of 70 percent extract three times daily.

Cayenne

Believed to be one of the best herbs for cardiovascular health, cayenne pepper contains capsaicin, which has been shown to lower cholesterol and triglycerides. It is also said to reduce blood clots, reduce blood pressure, and relieve pain. It may have some anti-cancer properties, as well. Just ½ teaspoon twice daily of cayenne pepper, added to a dish or to a Detox Blast Smoothie will help you feel better.

Your Body's pH

Why is eating an alkaline-rich diet so important for your health and well-being? Disease is the result of acid in the body, so an unhealthy lifestyle and poor eating habits can lead to illness. Even aches and pains can be the result of too much acidity in the body. Simply getting a massage or taking an aspirin for a headache may lead to temporary relief, but it won't heal the problem. Real healing comes from making changes in the foods you eat and the lifestyle choices you make. It is said that disease begins on the plate. Healthy foods and hydration will make your blood more alkaline.

The health of your body depends on the health of your cells, and your cells need oxygen, water, minerals (especially potassium, sodium, magnesium, calcium, and zinc), and the ability to eliminate their own waste. The quality of your blood affects the quality of your cells. In order for cells to be healthy, the blood must remain slightly alkaline. Blood alkalinity is measured on a scale of 0 to 14, with the low end of the scale acid, the middle neutral, and the upper end of the scale alkaline. In order for the blood to be a healthy environment for the cells, it must maintain a slightly alkaline pH of 6.0–8.0. You can test the pH of your foods and bodily fluids with litmus paper from any pharmacy or health food store.

When blood is acidic, red blood cells start to clump together. When that happens, they are no longer able to travel through the capillaries and feed the cells in the body. In order to keep cells healthy and slightly alkaline, it's essential to drink plenty of pure water and eat alkaline-rich foods. Test your drinking water to make sure it's alkaline, and definitely get a water filter for your sink if you are going to drink tap water. In addition to fruits and vegetables, pickles can help to alkalinize the body. They are an excellent digestive aid eaten with a meal, at the end of a meal, or as a snack. Pickles cured in sea salt are best for the body.

Alkaline-Forming Foods

Almonds
Asparagus
Avocados
Beet tops
Broccoli
Brussels sprouts
Cabbages
Carrots
Cauliflower
Celery
Coconuts
Cucumbers
Dates
Garlic
Green beans
Green leafy vegetables
Lima beans
Onions
Peppers (all colors)
Radishes
Spinach
Soybeans
Tofu
Turnip tops
Walnuts
Wheat grass

Acid-Forming Foods

Beef
Beer
Butter
Cheese
Chicken
Coffee
Eggs
Fish
Hot dogs
Lobster
Margarine
Mushrooms
Oysters
Pork
Refined sugars
Shrimp
Sour cream
Tea
Turkey
Veal
Whole wheat and rye breads
Wine
Yogurt

What about Candida?

Many people who eat unhealthy, acid-forming foods and live an acidic lifestyle of prescription drugs, excessive alcohol, caffeine, deficient exercise, lack of full spectrum light, chemical preservatives and pesticides, and stress suffer from candida.

So, what is it? Candida albicans is a form of yeast that normally resides in the gastrointestinal tract. Usually it lives in harmony with other microorganisms and performs a variety of important functions. However, when the body's pH becomes acidic, it overpopulates and becomes a parasitic fungus that attacks the weakest cells.

Some researchers think that candida may be the disease behind other diseases. Some of the most common symptoms of candida are bloating, abdominal aches and pains, headaches, migraines, and fatigue. Whenever you experience any kind of painful or uncomfortable condition, it's a good idea to ask your doctor to test for candida, as many mainstream doctors have yet to consider candida as a culprit for sickness.

The two main causes of candida are a diet high in sugar and the overuse of antibiotics. Taking acidophilus as a supplement (rather than through dairy products like yogurt) on a daily basis is an excellent defense against candida. The other best treatment for candida is to follow an alkaline-based diet, consisting of 70 to 80 percent fresh fruits, vegetables, and whole grains, and to eliminate refined sugars and processed foods. It may be necessary to also eliminate natural sugars like fruits as well until the candida growth has been stopped, and then to reintroduce them once symptoms have disappeared.

Additional Cleanses to Assist the Colon and Body

Colon Hydrotherapy

A colonic is not the most comfortable experience in the world—but it certainly isn't painful, and the benefits are powerful. Releasing excess waste from the colon is incredibly healing for the body, mind, and spirit. You will get used to the sensation and learn to relax during the treatment.

Decaying fecal matter in the colon creates an acidic environment that literally poisons the body. Even when you have no noticeable symptoms and feel perfectly healthy, it's still important to cleanse the colon and large intestines regularly to ensure lasting health and energy. If you aren't comfortable getting a colonic, then you'll find it beneficial to go through a salt water flush about four times a year instead (see page 42).

I realized how necessary regular colonics were when I learned these facts at a seminar:

- The average person has 7 to 25 pounds of fecal matter in his or her system.
- A constipated colon is generally lined with accumulated feces that becomes hardened and lodged

in the pockets of the wall. This fecal matter buildup can result in 5 to 15 pounds of added weight and can take many months or years to eliminate.

- Many people lose significant weight from regular colonics. Some overweight patients have eliminated as much as 10 to 25 pounds.
- The colon causes more disease than any other organ in the body. It is said to initiate 80 percent of all critical illnesses.

Parasite Cleanse

Although you may think you won't have parasites if you eat healthy foods, disease-causing parasites affect a large percentage of the population. Salt flushes and colonics can help to cleanse the colon and large intestine, but they don't necessarily exterminate parasites. The best way to get rid of parasites is with an herbal parasite cleanse at least once or twice a year.

There are hundreds of types of parasites that can live in the human body, such as hookworms, tapeworms, heartworms, and roundworms. Parasite eggs enter the human body through food, such as meat that isn't fully cooked or unwashed fruits and vegetables. They can also be water- or airborne or passed along by pets. Once they are inside the body, they can burrow into the lungs, liver, brain, or eyes, but the majority live inside the colon and the intestines. Because parasite eggs can live for only about 27 hours in the body, the cleaner your diet, the faster elimination will occur. This is why an easily digested plant-based diet is so important; fecal matter is less likely to build up in the body, giving parasites a place to lay their eggs. Meat and dairy products are much harder for the body to digest, and elimination time takes longer. Meat takes about three days to eliminate. While you are on the Fresh Fruit Cleanse, you'll notice how easily you eliminate, and that's because fruit is nature's purest and most water-rich food.

Here's an easy test to find out if you potentially have parasites: mix 2 tablespoons of sesame seeds in 8 ounces of water, and drink without chewing the seeds. Note the time of day you drank the mixture, and watch your bowel movements to see if the seeds were eliminated. If it takes more than 27 hours to eliminate all the seeds, there's a strong possibility your body has parasites.

Herbal Parasite Cleanses

The most common herbs used to eliminate parasites are black hull walnuts, wormwood, pumpkin seeds, cloves, and fennel seeds. Although there are no side effects from the herbs used in a parasite cleanse, your body may go through a "healing crisis" as it begins to eliminate the parasites. You may experience fatigue, bodily aches, or even a fever. If this happens, know this is the body's process of cleansing itself of toxic organisms. Eat only light food when experiencing symptoms like this—and symptoms or not, be sure to drink lots of water to continue flushing the toxins out of your body. You can find a parasite cleansing kit at any natural health food store.

Also, pumpkin seeds have been used by Native American cultures for centuries to eliminate parasites. Eating pumpkin seeds as a snack can help to deworm the body, as well.

For more information about herbal parasite cleanses, visit www.the-natural-path.com/parasite-cleanse.html.

Kidney Detox

The kidneys are extremely important to your overall health and well-being. Unhealthy, toxin-filled kidneys can contribute to low back pain and kidney stones and cause other health problems. The kidneys are located above the waistline and the hip, under a layer of muscle, on either side of your backbone. Cranberry juice is good for kidney health, but drinking Kidney Detox Juice while you're on the Fresh Fruit Cleanse and continuing with it afterward, for a total of three weeks, will strengthen the benefits of your cleansing experience and your overall well-being. And if you have any kidney stones, this formula will help your body dissolve them and pass them painlessly.

Kidney Detox Juice

Makes 1 serving

1 cup organic unfiltered apple juice (raw or unpasteurized is best)

20–30 drops hydrangea root tincture

Drink a full cup 3 or 4 times a day for 3 weeks.

Liver Detox

After the skin, the liver is the largest organ in the human body. The long-term effect of a toxic liver manifests itself in bloating and lethargy, allergies, weight gain, and premature aging, such as wrinkles and spotted, dry, and leathery skin. For the skin to be beautiful, the liver must be clean. One of the easiest ways to improve the health of the liver is to decrease consumption of alcohol and saturated fats.

Drinking this Liver Detox Tea is one of the simplest and tastiest ways to detoxify your liver. Lemon and ginger help to improve lymph and blood circulation, which cleanses the blood. Lemons are packed with enzymes that make them one of the most beneficial and restorative foods for the liver. You can purchase lemon ginger tea, but your own tea made with fresh ingredients is so much better for your health.

Liver Detox Tea

Makes 1 serving

juice of ¼–⅓ lemon

2 inches fresh ginger, peeled and chopped

stevia

Boil water and pour over lemon juice and chopped ginger in a mug. Sweeten with stevia, to taste.

Changing Your Diet for Good

The saying "you are what you eat" is true. The unhealthy effects of poor eating habits accumulate, and over time become evident physically, mentally, emotionally, and spiritually. When we are children, our bodies are much more resilient because there is no residue from years of unhealthy eating in the cells, blood, organs, and skin. But as we mature, the effects of years of poor eating and toxic lifestyle choices become obvious, and we begin to realize we must make changes if we want to feel, look, and be well. People who eat a healthy diet look and feel radiant.

> Take good care of your body. It's the only place you have to live.
>
> —*Jim Rohn, American entrepreneur, author, and motivational speaker (1930–2009)*

To feel good and to be healthy and beautiful, it's essential that you transform your way of living and undo the effects of years of unhealthy living. The key is to eat as much raw, life-filled, sun-rich food as possible—that is, fruits, vegetables, and whole grains. The changes you see from just a few days of cleansing with the Fresh Fruit Cleanse will inspire you to stay on the path of health and wellness and to make healthier choices for yourself, even after you cleanse. You may not make all of these changes at once, and, in fact, it's best to let it happen naturally as you are ready to make changes. You can progress on the path of wellness one day at a time. You don't have to give up everything all at once, and you don't have to give up something completely, unless it's a habit or addiction that's seriously impacting your health and well-being.

Vegetarianism

When I began yoga in 2002, I dated someone who was a vegetarian and I began to live a vegetarian lifestyle after that. As I progressed on the path of yoga, I found that many people who practice yoga are vegetarians, some for ethical reasons and some for health reasons.

For the last nine years I have eaten a mostly vegetarian diet, eating fish only occasionally. A couple of times during those years, I went months without eating fish at all, which was hard for me at the time. It was a good exercise for me to realize I could do it, but I think when we are really ready to make a lasting change in life, it doesn't feel like such a sacrifice. Nowadays, I find the healthier I eat, the less and less I desire meat and dairy.

If everyone ate a mostly plant-based diet and organic meat on occasion, the world would be a much healthier place. Factory farming puts excessive stress and strain on the planet and on our health, and unethical farming practices are perpetrated on animals all over the world. A diet rich in vegetables, fruits, and whole grains is healthiest for our bodies and would be healthiest for the planet as well.

Eating Meat

If you choose to eat meat, avoid consuming it with starches like bread and pasta in the same meal. The best starches to eat are healthy ones like brown rice, quinoa, and other whole grains, but it's still best to wait two hours to eat meat after consuming any kind of starch.

Eating meat between 10 a.m. and 4 p.m. is ideal, because this is when digestion is strongest and your body is best able to eliminate any waste load from the meat. It's also helpful to eat lots of vegetables when consuming meat, as the fiber in the vegetables absorbs any chemicals in the meat. Also, the antioxidants in vegetables help to protect the body from any cellular damage caused by the meat.

Spices will also help to neutralize parasites, which can be found in meat. Salt and pepper are not strong enough to cause this neutralization. It's important to use spices like garlic, oregano, rosemary, thyme, cloves, turmeric, cilantro, cumin, asafetida, ginger, and cayenne pepper. The meat should be smothered with spices to neutralize any parasitic effects; small amounts of spices are not enough. Examples of smothered meats are blackened fish or curried goat.

The Zigzag Method

What is the zigzag method? It's a way of living healthily but still letting yourself enjoy something that's not so healthy from time to time. When we realize the only real lasting joy comes through healthy living practices and meditation, then we can enjoy the pleasures of life, in moderation. With the zigzag method, you eat a healthy diet rich in fruits, vegetables, and whole grains five days a week and then let yourself enjoy more indulgent meals the other two days.

You might find the occasional indulgent meal or treat is also healing for your body, mind, and soul. Maybe it will remind you of growing up and sharing a special meal with someone you loved so much. In that moment, you'll remember how loved you are and that all is well in life. Deprivation or denial is not the answer. Eat healthily most of the time, but, let *all* food, in moderation, nourish you.

Vegan Recipes for a Healthy Life

These recipes are for after you finish the Fresh Fruit Cleanse, though you may be inspired to continue eating the recipes from the Fresh Fruit Cleanse Menu, too. All of the recipes in this book are good for your body, mind, and soul.

Breakfast

Banana Cream Pancakes

Makes 4 servings

1⅓ cups flour
1 tablespoon baking powder
½ teaspoon nutmeg
1½ cups light coconut milk
1 large ripe banana (about 1 cup, mashed)
1 teaspoon vanilla
coconut oil

In a large bowl combine the flour, baking powder, and nutmeg. Add the coconut milk, banana, and vanilla, and mix well by hand or with a mixer. Pour just enough oil in the pan to coat it, and heat over low to medium heat. Ladle batter into the pan. Cook one side several minutes until bubbles form, then flip and cook the other side for 1 to 2 minutes. Serve with agave nectar, maple syrup, or raw honey.

Breakfast Quinoa

Makes 4 servings

2 cups water

1 cup quinoa

⅓ cup raisins

¼ cup goji berries

½ cup toasted slivered almonds

1 teaspoon ground cinnamon

To cook the quinoa, boil the water. Once the water is boiling add the quinoa and cover, simmering on medium-low to medium heat until all of the water is absorbed. Remove from the heat and allow to stand covered for 5 minutes. Mix in the remaining ingredients and serve warm or chilled. This dish is also great with almond milk poured over the top.

Nut Mylk

Makes 4 servings

½ cup favorite nuts or seeds

3 cups water, divided

pinch of sea salt

½ teaspoon alcohol-free vanilla extract

Soak the nuts in 1 cup of water for 2 hours. Drain and add the remaining 2 cups of water, salt, and vanilla. Blend until smooth. Nut Mylk will keep in the refrigerator for 4 days.

Quinoa Fruit Salad

Makes 2 servings

1 medium green apple, chopped
1 cup cubed mango
1 cup blackberries or blueberries
1 cup cooked quinoa
⅓ cup pumpkin seeds
Sooo Delicious Cashew Cream (see below)
ground cinnamon

Combine the fruits, and toss with the quinoa and pumpkin seeds. Top with Sooo Delicious Cashew Cream and a sprinkle of cinnamon.

Sooo Delicious Cashew Cream

Makes 4 servings

2 cups raw unsalted cashews
1 cup water

Soak the cashews in the water for 1 hour. Blend the soaked nuts and water until creamy. Serve over your favorite fruit salad. The cashew cream will keep in the refrigerator for 4 days. This can be sweetened with agave nectar or raw honey.

Vegan Raw Cereal

Makes 2 servings

½ cup chia seeds
½ cup pumpkin seeds
½ cup hemp seeds
½ cup chopped apple
¼ cup raisins

Combine all ingredients, and pour Nut Mylk over the mixture. Or, add raw honey to sweeten.

Smoothies

Cacao and Strawberry Dream Smoothie

Makes 2 servings

1½ cups water

1 cup strawberries

¼ cup raw unsalted almonds, soaked

4–5 dates, pitted

½ teaspoon alcohol-free vanilla extract

¼ cup raw cacao powder

1 tablespoon agave nectar

Blend all ingredients until smooth. Substitute blueberries for strawberries, if desired.

Emerald Champagne

Makes 2 servings

2 cups pineapple juice

1–2 celery ribs, halved

ice (for consistency)

Blend all ingredients until frothy. This refreshing drink will last in the fridge for 3 days.

(Adapted with permission from the *Fruit Day Cookbook*, published by School of Metaphysics.)

Green Energy Drink

Makes 1 serving

1½ cups water

2 cups spinach

2 small cucumbers

1 bunch parsley

1 lemon

1 tablespoon freshly grated ginger

Juice or blend all ingredients and enjoy.

Power Protein Smoothie

Makes 2 servings

2 cups water

1 large banana

2 tablespoons almond butter

1 teaspoon hemp protein powder

1 teaspoon alcohol-free vanilla extract

2 tablespoons agave nectar or raw honey

Blend until smooth, and enjoy.

Soups

Butternut Squash Soup

Makes 4 servings

1 medium yellow or red onion

½ teaspoon freshly grated or minced ginger

3 cloves garlic, minced

2 cups cubed butternut squash

1 large potato, cubed

salt and pepper, to taste

Sauté the onion until tender. Add the ginger and garlic, and sauté a few more minutes. Add the squash, potato, and enough water to cover the squash. Bring to a boil, and reduce heat to a simmer until the vegetables are soft, about 30 minutes. Blend with a mixer or stick blender until smooth. Add salt and pepper (I like white pepper).

Tropical Black Bean Soup

Makes 4-6 servings

2½ cups water

1 (14-ounce) can light coconut milk

1 (14.5-ounce) can diced tomatoes

1 (4-ounce) can diced green or jalapeño chile peppers
1 (15-ounce) can black beans, rinsed well
salt and pepper

Place the water, coconut milk, tomatoes, and peppers in a saucepan, and bring to a boil. Add the beans, cover the saucepan, and turn the heat off. Allow to sit for 3 to 5 minutes. Season to taste and serve. You can top with mango, salsa, avocado, or all three. This soup is so good and simple to make.

Sweet Potato Soup

Makes 4 servings

2 large sweet potatoes, peeled and cut in chunks
2 tablespoons light oil such as canola, extra virgin olive, or coconut
1½ tablespoons freshly grated ginger
½ teaspoon cayenne pepper, to taste
¾ cup light or regular coconut milk
2½ cups vegetable stock
chopped chives or cilantro, to taste, for garnish

Boil the sweet potatoes in water for about 15 minutes, or until very tender. Drain and set aside. Add the oil to a large pot on medium heat. Add the ginger, and sauté for a few minutes until fragrant. Add the cayenne pepper. Mix the sweet potatoes with the ginger and pepper. Add the coconut milk and 2 cups of the vegetable stock, and let cook for a few minutes. Blend (in a blender or using a stick blender) until smooth. Most likely, it will be more like a purée than a soup. Add vegetable stock until you get desired consistency. Garnish with chives or cilantro before serving.

Vegetable Soup

Makes 6 servings

1 medium yellow or red onion, chopped
2 carrots, chopped
2 celery ribs, chopped
6 cups vegetable stock
1 (14.5-ounce) can diced tomatoes
3 tablespoons chopped fresh basil or 1½ teaspoons dried
3 tablespoons chopped fresh parsley or 1½ teaspoons dried
3 tablespoons chopped fresh oregano or 1½ teaspoons dried
2 medium zucchini or other summer squash, sliced
1 bunch broccoli, cut into small florets
1 potato, boiled and diced (optional)
salt and pepper, to taste

Sauté the onion, carrots, and celery until tender. Add the vegetable stock, and bring to a boil. Turn down to simmer. Stir in the tomatoes and herbs, and simmer for 10 minutes. Add the zucchini, broccoli, and potato, if using, and cook another 5 to 10 minutes, or until tender. Season with salt and pepper. You can also add garlic, spinach, kale, or other vegetables—whatever you like will work. A can of beans, such as cannellini, is also a delicious addition.

Entrées

Asian Cole Slaw

Makes 4 servings

2 tablespoons agave nectar
¼ cup rice vinegar
salt and pepper, to taste
3 cups raw veggies or 1 package shredded cabbage or broccoli slaw

Whisk together the agave and vinegar, and season with salt and pepper. Add to the vegetables, toss well, and refrigerate.

Okra Creole

Makes 4–6 servings

½ yellow onion, chopped
1 rib celery, cut in ¼-inch slices
8 cups diced tomatoes
Creole seasoning
8 cups sliced okra, cut in ¼-inch pieces
1 green or red bell pepper, seeded and chopped

In a large saucepan, sauté the onion and celery in a little oil. Add the tomatoes and Creole seasoning, to taste. Simmer about 15 minutes. Stir in the okra and pepper. Cover and simmer another 15 minutes, stirring occasionally.

(Adapted with permission from the *Fruit Day Cookbook*, published by School of Metaphysics.)

Perfectly Pure Pizza

Makes 1 serving

1 (8.5-inch) sprouted grain tortilla
olive oil
spinach
heirloom tomato slices
mushrooms, sliced
red onion, diced
fresh basil leaves, chopped
tomato sauce or paste
balsamic vinegar

Heat the oven to 350°F. Brush the entire tortilla with olive oil, cover it in foil (to keep from getting crisp), and warm up in the oven or toaster oven. Brush tomato sauce or paste on the wrap if desired, and place the vegetables and basil on top. Drizzle with balsamic vinegar and heat in the oven until warm. The spinach may get a little crisp but will still be delicious.

Roasted Sweet Potatoes and Macadamia Nuts

Makes 4 servings

3 sweet potatoes, peeled and cubed

1 tablespoon olive oil

⅓ cup chopped macadamia nuts

4 cups spinach leaves

Dressing

1 tablespoon apple cider vinegar

1 teaspoon Dijon mustard

2 tablespoons macadamia nut oil

sea salt and pepper

Heat the oven to 375°F. Put the sweet potatoes in a bowl, and toss with olive oil. Place on a baking sheet, and bake for 10 minutes. Add the nuts to the sweet potatoes, and bake for another 10 minutes. Meanwhile, mix the dressing, seasoning it to taste. Place the sweet potatoes in a bowl, add the spinach and the dressing, and toss well.

Marinated Mixed Vegetables

Makes 4 servings

1 medium eggplant, sliced

½ cup mushrooms, sliced

1 (½-pound) bunch thin asparagus spears

1 red bell pepper, seeded and cut into strips

Marinade

½ cup soy sauce

¼ cup balsamic vinegar

1 tablespoon olive oil

1 tablespoon agave nectar

Heat the oven to 400°F. Layer the veggies in a dish with a small amount of water covering the bottom. Cook for 10 to 15 minutes, and drain if necessary. Meanwhile, mix the marinade. Toss the veggies with the marinade, and roast another 5 minutes. Serve over rice or your favorite grain, and top with pine nuts, if desired.

Tofu Hero Sandwich

Makes 4 servings

Tofu

1 package extra firm organic tofu, sliced into ¼–½-inch slabs
1 tablespoon olive oil
1 clove garlic, minced
¼ cup soy sauce
pepper, to taste

Sandwich

8 slices sprouted grain bread
½ cucumber, sliced
2 cups spinach leaves
1 medium tomato, sliced
4 slices vegan cheese
1 yellow bell pepper, seeded and sliced into rings
mushrooms, sliced, to taste
ground Dijon mustard

Heat the oven to 375°F. Layer the tofu in a glass baking dish. Mix the oil, garlic, soy sauce, and pepper. Pour the mixture over the tofu, then turn the tofu to coat it well. Bake for 20 minutes, turning once at 10 minutes. Spread mustard on the bread (you can toast it or not). Assemble the sandwiches with the ingredients however you wish.

Dressings

Lemon Vinaigrette

Makes 4 servings

½ cup extra-virgin olive oil or carrot juice
3 tablespoons fresh lemon juice
1 tablespoon fresh thyme or 1 teaspoon dried
1 tablespoon chopped fresh dill or 2 teaspoons dried
1 tablespoon chopped fresh chives or 2 teaspoons dried
ground rock salt, to taste
freshly ground pepper, to taste

Whisk together the ingredients, seasoning with salt and pepper

Good All-Ways Salad Dressing

Makes 8 servings

1 cup vegetable oil
⅓ cup olive oil
1 cup apple cider vinegar
½ cup fresh lemon juice
1 tablespoon salt
½ tablespoon pepper
½ tablespoon celery seed
¼ tablespoon dried rosemary
3 tablespoons minced garlic
1 tablespoon dried oregano
⅛ tablespoon dried thyme
½ tablespoon dried basil
1 tablespoon dried parsley

Mix all the ingredients together. Let the mixture sit in the refrigerator for 12 hours to fully release the flavors. Shake, serve, and enjoy. This dressing is good on salads, greens, pastas, and stir-fries.

(Adapted with permission from the *Fruit Day Cookbook*, published by School of Metaphysics.)

Desserts

Banana Cinnamon Buttermylk

Makes 4 servings

1 large banana

1 teaspoon ground cinnamon

¼ cup Sooo Delicious Cashew Cream (see page 192)

1½–2 cups water

Blend until creamy. Substitute almond butter for cashew cream, if desired.

Banana Fruit Salad Parfait

Makes 2 servings

2 medium bananas, sliced

½ cup strawberries, chopped

½ cup blueberries

1 tablespoon hemp seeds (optional)

1 tablespoon sunflower seeds (optional)

Layer the fruits with Sooo Delicious Cashew Cream or any other nut cream. Top with seeds, if desired.

Booty Shakin' Good Chocolate

Makes 6–8 servings

⅓ cup melted cacao butter

¼ cup agave nectar

¼ teaspoon alcohol-free vanilla extract

pinch of sea salt

½ cup raw cacao powder, sifted

Mix the melted cacao butter with the agave, vanilla, and sea salt in a warm bowl. Slowly mix in the raw cacao powder until the mixture is smooth. You can add the mixture into a small ice cube tray to make pieces of chocolate.

Peach or Apple Pistachio Cobbler

Makes 4 servings

Filling

4 cups apples or peaches, or both, chopped

2 tablespoons maple syrup

1 tablespoon alcohol-free vanilla extract

Crust topping

½ cup raw, unsalted pistachios

¼ teaspoon sea salt

½ cup pitted Medjool dates

Combine all the filling ingredients in a bowl and mix well. To make the crust, combine the pistachios and salt in a food processor, and pulse into medium-sized pieces. Add the dates, and process until crumbly. In small dishes, spoon the crust topping over the filling, and serve. The cobbler will keep in the refrigerator for 2 days.

Pumpkin Pie

Makes 6–8 servings

1 (15-ounce) can pumpkin purée (not pumpkin pie purée)

1 cup rice milk

¾ cup agave nectar

¼ cup potato or cornstarch

1 tablespoon maple syrup

1 teaspoon vanilla extract

1 teaspoon ground cinnamon

½ teaspoon ground ginger

¼ teaspoon ground nutmeg or allspice

1 organic spelt, gluten-free, or vegan pie crust from the freezer section

Heat the oven to 425°F. Blend all the filling ingredients until smooth. Taste it to make sure you like the flavor—you may want to add a little more maple syrup, for example. Pour the mixture into the pie crust. Bake for 10 minutes. Then turn the oven down to 350°F, and continue to bake for 50 minutes. Let the pie cool to room temperature, and put it in the refrigerator to chill overnight. If fresh pumpkin is available, you can use it (you'll need 1¾ cups). For a creamier pie, use light or regular coconut milk instead of rice milk.

Raw Nut Brownies

Makes 16 (2 x 2-inch) squares

2 cups raw walnuts, chopped
1 cup raw pecans, chopped
4 tablespoon water
½ cup raw cacao powder
1 teaspoon alcohol-free vanilla extract
22 dates, pitted and chopped
1 tablespoon agave nectar

Place all ingredients in a mixer, and blend until smooth. It's also helpful to use a dough blender. Spoon out thick mixture into a 8 x 8-inch square baking pan, and press firmly. Refrigerate for 2 hours, and serve.

Tofu & Mixed Berry Cheesecake

Makes 6–8 servings

Crust

¾ cup Earth Balance buttery spread
2 cups graham cracker crumbs (I like Mi-Del brand)

Filling

1 (12-ounce) package silken tofu (from sprouted soybeans)
1 cup non-dairy cream cheese (I like Tofutti brand)
1 tablespoon olive or coconut oil
¼ cup maple syrup plus 2 teaspoons for topping
¼ rice or soy milk
2 teaspoons arrowroot

1 tablespoon vanilla extract

1 teaspoon lemon extract

1–2 cups fresh berries

Heat the oven to 350°F. Spray an 8- or 9-inch round baking pan with organic canola oil. To make the crust, melt the Earth Balance in a medium saucepan, turn off the heat, and mix in the graham cracker crumbs. Press the mixture into the bottom and sides of baking pan, and bake for 5 minutes. Combine all the filling ingredients except the berries with a mixer. Pour the filling into the crust, and bake for 45 minutes to 1 hour. Let cool to room temperature. Mix the berries with 2 teaspoons of maple syrup, and top the cheesecake. Chill overnight.

14

Releasing Yourself from the Toxic Western Life

The traditional Western diet and lifestyle is toxic, and has been for decades. Conventional produce is laced with harmful pesticides, foods in our grocery stores are processed with chemicals and artificial ingredients, and a fast food lifestyle full of unhealthy fats, salts, and sugars has overwhelmed our nation and the world.

How did we find ourselves at a toxic dinner table? How did we arrive at this terrifying diet?

There was a time when we valued simple living, and our food came directly from the earth and from farms in our local communities. When industrialization swept the nation, the organic farming culture of the past several hundred years began to die away. Americans left their homes to go to cities to find work and care for their families. The American way of eating and living changed. Manufacturing soon made an impact on the foods we were eating.

We began to fill our homes—and our bodies—with artificial, processed, and frozen foods. Over the years, an ever-increasing number of fast food outlets sprouted, filling us with the same unhealthy fats and artificial ingredients when we were away from home.

During the last decade, we've gradually woken up. Whole food nutrition and natural, organic eating is making its way back into our kitchens, grocery stores, and restaurants. Yes, there's still fast food on many street corners and plenty of artificial foods in grocery stores, but we are remembering there was a time when we ate and lived simply, naturally, and healthily from the earth, rather than from processed, chemical-laden foods.

Cleanse Your Home

Many people believe the best practice is to eat foods that are as closely connected to the sun as possible, mainly fresh fruits and vegetables. When that's not possible, then it's best to eat natural, organic, unprocessed foods. If you have anything that is processed and filled with artificial substances and chemicals in your pantry, refrigerator, or freezer, throw it out.

Although it may not be so easy to change the unhealthy ways of the whole world, we can change our inner world, where real change always begins. The first step to getting healthy is eliminating unhealthy foods from your home. Before you do the Fresh Fruit Cleanse, be sure to cleanse your home of any unhealthy foods. Eliminate foods high in salt, refined sugar, or refined grains, or containing artificial ingredients. If it's not natural, stop eating it—and get it out of your home.

Be Honest

If you are struggling with any addiction, whether it's food, alcohol, nicotine, caffeine, shopping, or anything else, the first step is to be honest with yourself and to acknowledge your struggle. Sometimes we don't realize the addictions controlling us. For a long time, I would justify unhealthy habits and behaviors for many different reasons. At some point, I finally realized that I had a problem and needed to change my ways.

The Fresh Fruit Cleanse will help you make positive changes in your life. For most of us it's a process. Each time you cleanse, you will realize what unhealthy habits or behaviors are controlling you and your life. Over time, cleansing will help you find balance and moderation in all your choices. If you used to drink half a bottle of wine every night, and after cleansing you drink only a few glasses a week, that's an improvement. If you used to drink a cup of coffee a day, and after cleansing you have just a couple of cups a week, that's progress. Celebrate yourself and the positive changes you are making with positive and healthy rewards like a trip to the spa, a pedicure, or a relaxing retreat by yourself or with a friend.

Identify Your Dependencies

Actually identifying a dependency and accepting that you're in its grip is key to getting rid of it. It's one thing to acknowledge a habit, but accepting that you may need professional help to change is another step altogether. If your habits and choices are significantly damaging your life, this may be a step you need to take. Or, since environment is stronger than will, you may need to change your environment and surround yourself with healthier people and friends who share your aspirations and visions for health and well-being.

Caffeine

There is some belief that the antioxidants in coffee may help protect the human body from such conditions as premature aging, cardiovascular disease, and certain cancers. However, like anything, it is best consumed in moderation.

Because caffeine is a mild diuretic, excessive use (more than 3 cups of coffee per day) can cause of bone mineral density loss. This happens because caffeine speeds up the urination cycle, leaching calcium, which is lost through urine. It's believed long-term caffeine use can lead to the development of osteoporosis. Caffeine also increases the heart rate, which causes restlessness, anxiety, and sleeplessness. While moderate caffeine use may be OK for some people, caffeine is highly addictive. A healthy lifestyle, good nutrition, and regular exercise are able to provide all the energy you need.

Try starting off your day with a piece of fresh fruit or a fruit smoothie instead of coffee. Fruits are among the most naturally energizing foods in the world, and they'll kick-start your day as well as satisfy your hunger and thirst and keep you going for hours.

Sugar and Fat

You might not think of food as an addiction, but it is. I have been addicted to many foods in my life, and the list is too long to name them all here. I really craved the unhealthy sugars and fats in those foods. In fact, most people aren't addicted to actual foods but to the added sugars and saturated fats in them. As you eat a store-bought, processed pizza or a piece of chocolate layer cake, think about how much sugar and fat have gone into them to make them palatable. Then savor a juicy organic orange or mango and know that you're getting pure, wholesome food with natural sweetness and practically no fat. The fruit is delicious, and you won't feel bloated after you've eaten.

I didn't come to the realization overnight that fruit is better for me and tastier than those sugary, fatty foods, but I now firmly believe it. Over the last ten years, I've gradually been able to heal and transform my relationship with food through the Fresh Fruit Cleanse, healthy living, exercise, and yoga. I no longer live to eat, I now eat to live.

Alcohol

Alcohol abuse is one of the major causes of social, economic, and public health problems in our country. Excessive alcohol damages the liver and other organs, is a depressant, and can cause weight gain. Too much alcohol can also contribute to high blood pressure, heart failure, stroke, fetal alcohol syndrome in pregnancy, and certain cancers, as well as injury and death.

When abused, alcohol is destructive to a person's body, mind, and spirit and it is discouraged on any spiritual path to well-being. While an occasional glass of wine is OK for many people, as you progress on a healthier path you may find you desire alcohol less. The Fresh Fruit Cleanse is an excellent way to experience life without alcohol—and the more often you cleanse, the more you may realize you can do without it.

Nicotine

If you are addicted to nicotine, I understand your struggle—but, if you are smoking cigarettes, stop! I started smoking at the age of 13, and if I could stop, I know you can, too. Smoking is one of the worst things you can do for your health. Most of us know the hazardous side effects of smoking. It causes numerous health problems, including lung cancer as well as cancers of the lip, larynx, esophagus, pancreas, cervix, bladder, and kidneys. Smoking can also cause emphysema, heart attacks, underweight newborn children, miscarriages, strokes, cataracts, and impotence. Also, nothing ages the body more than smoking.

If, like me, you have been a smoker for a long time, quitting may be the hardest thing you ever do. However, with the positive changes you'll experience with the Fresh Fruit Cleanse, you'll definitely know it's possible.

Healing: One Day at a Time

If you can't see yourself living happily without alcohol, your favorite junk food, or something else, there's a good chance you are physically, mentally, or emotionally dependent on it. The Fresh Fruit Cleanse will help you let go of unhealthy habits and cravings by being aware of the emotional trigger behind them. The moment you choose to make a healthier choice instead of giving into the craving is the moment you begin to heal yourself from its power over you. Once you understand why you are doing something unhealthy, you will be able to let go of it, one day at a time. You are only really free from something when you no longer need it to feel better. For a long time I couldn't imagine being able to live without alcohol or certain foods in my life. But, as I have progressed on the path of wellness, I have found I feel best when I make healthier choices for myself.

The path of health is not a path of denial—it's a path of making choices that allow you to feel your best. As you gain control over your choices through the Fresh Fruit Cleanse and other healthy practices, you will feel empowered to do what's best for your life. No longer will temptation control you; you will rise above it. Anything is possible when you realize the only day you need to focus on making better choices is today. Let go of worrying about tomorrow. Making a healthier choice today will lead you into a happier, healthier, and better tomorrow.

Healing the Past

To be able to focus clearly, you must resolve any psychological distractions that caused you to neglect your body, mind, or spirit in the first place. The Fresh Fruit Cleanse is an incredibly powerful process for recognizing and then healing the emotional and mental triggers that caused you to make unhealthy choices.

Often, unhealthy desires come from not feeling good about yourself. It's surreal to think that we can carry feelings of fear or shame from childhood experiences into adult years and that those feelings can cause us to make poor choices. Many people have dealt with some kind of physical, verbal, emotional, or sexual mistreatment or abuse. Until the wounds from those experiences are healed, they will play themselves out in relationships, including relationship with food. It's important to understand how experiences in life have affected us and how they impact the way we treat ourselves and others.

Feel to Heal

It is said that almost all feelings about life experiences are kept in the emotional storehouse of the body, which is connected to the reproductive organs, also known as the second chakra (energy center) in yoga. The emotion doesn't have to stem from something as traumatic as verbal or sexual abuse. We can store unfelt or unresolved emotions about something seemingly insignificant, such as the shame of getting a B instead of an A on a test or wearing the same outfit as someone else to a party. Or perhaps it's something hurtful the bully down the street said to you when you were a child. Emotions from some kind of physical pain or trauma may also be stored.

One of the reasons yoga is so awesome is because it encourages you to feel your emotions so you can release them in a healthy way and heal past hurts. As you go through the poses, you feel places in your body where you have held onto some kind of physical, mental, or emotional tension—and you can let that tension go. Feeling to heal is about learning how to release emotions in a healthy way instead of taking them out on someone else. Many times, I've screamed, laughed, and cried as I felt something in a pose. Yoga, like the Fresh Fruit Cleanse, can release the flow of blocked energy or emotions in the body to allow feelings to flow and healing to happen.

Your task is not to seek for love, but merely to seek and find all the barriers in yourself you have built against it.

—*Rumi*

Anytime I was using alcohol or drugs as a way to connect with others, it wasn't a true connection. That's only possible when we allow ourselves to be completely exposed and can let go of hiding behind fear. If there are any places in yourself where you don't feel good about the person you are, let go of hiding in those places. One of my greatest teachers says that, *our greatest fear is the fear of being seen.* Now, there is nothing in my life that I'm afraid of anyone knowing. I realize I am loved and accepted no matter what, and so are you. If you are afraid you won't be loved because of something that's happened in your life, find a supportive friend, family member, or counselor to tell.

Your Thoughts Can Heal You

My first yoga teacher introduced me to the work of Louise L. Hay, a leader in the self-improvement movement for the last 40 years. One of her books is *Heal Your Body,* a guide to loving yourself and healing your body and life through the practice of positive thought patterns and affirmations. She and many others believe aging, as well as a high percentage of diseases, are psychosomatic and are caused by stress. Her book is wonderful, and I've consulted it many times to help heal even the most minor physical ailment. To learn more about Louise Hay, you can visit her website (www.louisehay.com) or purchase her book.

Change Is Good

Going through the Fresh Fruit Cleanse gives you the opportunity to fully comprehend where and why you are making unhealthy choices and how you can remedy the situation. Realize, though, as you begin to make changes in life, things around you will change. Allow any changes that are good for you to happen. Surrender yourself to God's plan for you. I've found that as you grow on the spiritual path and make better choices for yourself, in time unhealthy habits and behaviors just fall away. Old desires and cravings fade. If you need to let go of any unhealthy relationships, don't be afraid to—but also don't give up hope that some relationships might grow healthier in time. While it may not happen overnight, as you become healthier, the people around you just might grow healthier, too.

Love is giving someone the space to evolve.

—*Michael Brown, spiritual teacher and author*

Let go of worrying about how long it takes others to change, and focus on growing healthier, better, and stronger every day with the support of loved ones and friends. The greatest thing you can do, besides grow and be well yourself, is to love and pray for the people around you whom you wish to see happy and healthy. Love everyone in your life equally, including your neighbors, friends, family, partners, and even people you have felt challenged to love. God's grace and love and good people around you in life are all you need.

Sometimes, though, people make positive changes in their lives and then find it's difficult to stay on a healthy path. If you fall back into unhealthy habits, it doesn't mean you are a failure. It means you are human. Any time you feel as if you've strayed from the path, you can get back on again. Just take it one day at a time. Remind yourself you are doing the best you can, and commit to doing and being better, no matter how long it takes.

Visualization

My first yoga teacher would often tell her weight-loss story. When she was overweight, she was inspired to look like and exude the beauty and strength of a fitness model she had seen on a magazine cover. By continuously visualizing herself the way she wanted to look, feel, and be, she gradually transformed into that image she had of herself. The reality is the mind and willpower are very strong, and you have unlimited potential to attract good things to yourself and others around you through positive thoughts and visualization.

> All that you are is a result of what you have thought. Mind is everything. What you think you become.
>
> —*Buddha*

Perhaps you also have a mental image of how you would like to look and feel. Before you begin the Fresh Fruit Cleanse, visualize yourself as the healthy, beautiful, strong, energetic, and radiant person you wish to be. If you keep focusing your mind in a positive way and making healthy choices, you will evolve into that beautiful and healthy vision of yourself.

Awakening Your Willpower

> The opposite of willpower isn't won't power, it's addiction.
>
> —*Paramahansa Yogananda*

Food can be a drug that has tremendous power over the mind. Many people use food as a drug to numb, comfort, distract, or manage emotional distress. What's so powerful about the Fresh Fruit Cleanse is that, at the moment you are tempted to eat something unhealthy that will weigh you down, you can look into your mind, observe your cravings, and recognize the real cause behind them. If you are addicted to a certain food, you will begin to realize why you are addicted to it. In that moment, you gain real power over something that previously had control over you, and instead of giving in you decide to make a healthier choice.

Did you know that researchers conducted a study in which half of the participants lifted weights and the other half just thought about lifting weights? The people who lifted weights increased their strength by 30 percent, and the ones who just thought about it increased their strength by 22 percent. Many studies like this prove the power our thoughts and minds have over our own bodies and selves, and everything around us, too. As you realize the true power of your thoughts, you have a spiritual responsibility to exercise your mind in a positive way for the benefit of yourself and the world around you.

Your Health Is Your Wealth

An old proverb says that health is wealth. Health is the greatest blessing there is. When you feel healthy, everything in life becomes better and God can bless your life in amazing ways. Many people wonder how they can afford a healthier lifestyle. The truth is you can't afford not to be healthy. The healthier you are, the more connected you will be to God's light and life force itself, and you will feel strengthened and inspired in all aspects of your life.

Yes, you can afford to be healthy. As your lifestyle grows healthier, you will find you eat out less often, so it's a matter of reevaluating and redistributing your budget. You are worth an investment in yourself, but you must believe you are. You can afford to buy healthy supplements, like spirulina and maca, and the foods you need to feel your best. Commit to yourself and the Fresh Fruit Cleanse, and you will see you are provided for and that you are attracting good into your life.

> Physiological changes may even be made to occur in the body by willpower. There is no time element involved; place a thought in the mind and hold it there, and think that the thing is done and your whole body and mind will respond to it. Nor does it take time to acquire or discard a habit if you exercise sufficient willpower. It is all in your mind.
>
> *—Paramahansa Yogananda*

Through cleansing, healthy nutrition, and conscious living practices like yoga and meditation, you will realize that anything is possible. Not only will you be able to cleanse for three, five, or seven days, or however long you choose, but you will be strengthened to realize anything you are meant to do or be in life. You will be able lose weight, get in shape, heal, awaken radiant joy and beauty, and transform yourself and your life in positive ways, because you will know that you can become anything you focus your heart and mind on. Pour your heart into what you are passionate about and you will prosper.

15

Life Practices: Changing the Little Things

Happiness lies, first of all, in health.

—George William Curtis,
American writer and public speaker (1824-1892)

Skin Care

I recently read a book called *Do You Have the Guts to Be Beautiful?* by Dr. Mitra Ray, Ph.D., and Jennifer Daniels, M.D., who advocate Juice Plus+® nutritional supplements, which I have taken for many years (see page 221). The authors reveal many secrets to beautiful and healthy skin, such as a cleansing facial made from rice bran, liquid vitamin C, lemon juice, and grapeseed oil. I had been using an unnatural soap for almost 20 years of my life but stopped after reading their book.

Of course, the healthier you eat, the better your skin will be. The Detox Blast Smoothie and the Green Protein Smoothie will give you a healthy, glowing complexion. Milk thistle is an ingredient in the Green Protein Smoothie, but feel free to add it to any other smoothie or your favorite juice to make your skin even better.

Papaya or mango facials are also wonderful. Simply peel either fruit, remove the seeds, and mix the flesh into a paste in a blender or food processor. Rub the papaya or mango paste on your face and leave it for 10 to 15 minutes before washing it off. Both fruits are excellent for removing clogged pores and hydrating the skin.

For the healthiest and most beautiful skin, I suggest reducing or eliminating all of the following items:

- Tobacco, coffee, black tea, and alcohol
- Over-the-counter medications, including pain killers, laxatives, sleeping pills, and cold and flu remedies
- Animal products (meat, fish, fowl, wild game, eggs, and cheese, butter, and other dairy)
- All beverages except good, clean water
- Sugarless chewing gums and breath mints
- Processed and packaged foods

I now use only natural skin-care products on my face and body. Here are my favorites:

Face:

- Freshly squeezed lemon juice rubbed on the face and forehead
- Kiehl's Acai Damage-Repairing Serum
- Chag-o-Power Skin Cream (available on amazon.com)

Body:

- Body Butter by Simple Apothecary
- Any all-natural body wash

Teeth:

- Tom's of Maine Fluoride-Free Toothpaste (available at any natural grocery store)

Abhyanga

One of the most wonderful techniques for your health is abhyanga, a form of self-care and massage from the ancient yet timeless practice of Ayurveda. Simply massage sesame oil or coconut oil all over your body first thing in the morning. And oil rubbed on the nasal passages will keep the sinus passages moisturized and help alleviate any sinus problems or congestion. Then perform your morning ritual, whether that's practicing yoga, exercising, meditating, or drinking a smoothie.

Afterward, take a shower and allow all the healing, medicinal, moisturizing benefits of the oil to be absorbed into the pores as they open up in the warmth of the shower. Abhyanga is also very helpful in protecting against airborne illnesses when flying, though it's best to shower to remove the odor of the oil before an airplane trip. But when flying on long international flights, consider leaving the oil on to keep your skin fully hydrated and protected.

Skin Brushing

Skin brushing is incredibly beneficial for health and well-being. A few of the benefits of skin brushing include enhancing the texture of your skin, promoting cell renewal, improving circulation, evening out fat deposits, lessening the appearance of cellulite and increasing muscle tone, and rejuvenating the nervous system. The lymphatic system is just below the outer surface of the skin and carries nutrients to and from the cells, helping to eliminate toxins from the cells. Because the lymphatic system is just below the surface of the skin, dry brushing is an effective way to stimulate circulation in the lymph vessels, which helps to accentuate the body's cleansing process and remove dead cells. It's especially effective before a bath or sauna. Brush your skin, using small circular strokes, starting from your limbs and working your way toward your heart. You can find a dry bristle brush at any health food store.

Water: The Life Blood of Everything

Let's talk about water. Over the last ten years, bottled water has swept our country and the world. There's a widespread belief that bottled water is better than tap water, and it's true that some high-quality bottled waters are. However, bottled water isn't the healthiest option. Aside from the harmful chemicals found in water bottles, the simple act of bottling changes the water from its natural state. The water has been heated or cooked, pressed through a very small filter, or treated by ultraviolet light. All of these processes scramble the natural molecular structure of the water and change the natural state of the water from the way Mother Nature intended it to be.

The healthiest water for you is spring water, which comes directly from the earth. However, most bottled spring waters aren't from natural springs but from wells. There are a few exceptions, like Mountain Valley Spring Water, but your best bet is to go directly to the source. To find out the location of a natural spring near you, visit www.findaspring.com. Be sure to fill and store the spring water in glass bottles. You'll love the taste of spring water, and cooking with it improves the taste and quality of food.

If you can't locate good spring water, you're better off drinking filtered tap water, not bottled water, even though filters aren't able to eliminate unhealthy chemicals. And don't forget a water filter for your shower—the high level of chlorine in most tap water is very damaging to skin and hair, and it kills healthy along with unhealthy bacteria in the intestines.

Sunlight

Sunlight is very important to your health, and it's even a form of nourishment since it provides your body with vitamin D. One of the best ways to reenergize is to spend 10 to 15 minutes in the sun each day. Sunlight helps to produce serotonin, the feel-good chemical in the brain, and helps to ward off depression. In fact, many health experts believe sunlight may prevent more cancers than it causes.

Nutritional Supplements

I've been taking Juice Plus+® for nine years, and it's the best whole food supplement I've found. Although not a replacement for fresh fruits and vegetables, it is one of the best ways to give your body increased vitamins and minerals from whole food nutrition. Juice Plus+® capsules are filled with real fruits and vegetables that have been juiced, freeze dried, and pulverized into a powder. The capsules don't provide any fiber, which is one of the things that makes fruits and vegetables so good for you, but they do provide all of the nutrients you need. Most people don't get the recommended daily value of vitamins and minerals. Juice Plus+® helps you build a stronger nutritional foundation with mega amounts of vitamins A, C, and E in each serving. I find it so easy to take just two fruit capsules in the morning and two vegetable capsules in the evening, and because they're capsules I never tire of the taste. And a month's supply is affordable. To order Juice Plus+® capsules or to learn more about them, visit www.juiceplus.com/+lh88526.

> The body requires certain elements for its sustenance, but a good many people omit at least some of these elements from their diet every day. That is the reason why disease has uncontrolled sway everywhere. God did not create disease. Man creates it through continued wrong living. The cells are constantly decaying, and for that reason the body needs proper repairing with the right kind of food materials for new cell growth and maintenance. Every day the tissues should be supplied with the right kind of body building materials.
>
> —*Paramahansa Yogananda*

Of course, you can try other products, but they should be natural, whole food supplements. The most important thing is to avoid synthetic supplements. There is no evidence that pharmaceutically made vitamins and minerals are beneficial to your health, and there's even some belief that they can cause cancer. No matter what natural supplements you choose, make sure to eat a healthy amount of fresh fruits, vegetables, super foods, and whole grains every day, too.

Exercise

If you want to lose weight, stay in shape, look your best, and feel your best, then exercise is essential. Whatever you choose to do—walk, hike, bike, rollerblade, or work out on the elliptical—it's important to get a good cardiovascular workout for at least 30 minutes three times a week. If you practice yoga, you'll find you can alternate the days you work out and the days you do yoga. Although you can get a cardiovascular workout from yoga, that's not its true intention. It's meant to be a meditative practice for the total health of your body, mind, and spirit.

A few of the benefits of regular exercise include better mental and emotional health, prevention of chronic diseases (such as high blood pressure, cholesterol, diabetes, and some cancers), maintenance of a healthy weight, increased energy, better sleep, and an improved sex life. Let's not forget fun—I love spending time outdoors with friends and meeting people at the gym!

16

Yoga

According to yoga, we suffer because we live in ignorance. We are ignorant of our real nature. Our true nature lies beyond the restrictions of our careworn and humdrum existence, ecstatically free and untouched by suffering. Deep within the mind, beyond the faintest flicker of thought, it is experienced as an undying and omnipresent vastness. It is absolute consciousness. Animating everything in creation, this is the source and goal of all life.

—*The Yoga Sutras of Patanjali*,
translated and introduced by Alistair Shearer

In the West, most people think of yoga as a system of poses for acquiring physical fitness and mental well-being, but it is so much more than that. Yoga is a vehicle that helps you to grow in the best way possible and be the best you can be physically, mentally, emotionally, and spiritually. Yoga has inspired me to grow healthily in every area of life because it affects the choices I make, including the food I eat, the people I surround myself with, the way I love and am inspired to give, the work I do, my gratitude for life, and my faith in God.

The first stone-carved recordings of yoga are from around 3000 BC, and while its history is ancient, its benefits are timeless. People now are increasingly realizing how powerful this time-tested practice of health and well-being really is. Anyone of any shape, any age, and any size can do yoga. It's never too late to start, and no matter when you begin practicing yoga, you will realize awesome benefits for your body, mind, and spirit.

Physical Benefits

What makes yoga so powerful?

First, the poses are ingeniously designed to optimally align the muscular, skeletal, nervous, and internal organ systems of the body. All of the poses focus on keeping the internal body, nerves, glands, and organs healthy, as well as promote strong, toned muscles and a flexible, youthful body. A popular saying is that you are as young as your spine is flexible. This is why many of the yoga poses focus on the health of the spine and keeping it fluid and mobile.

The stimulation of the glands, particularly in forward bends, twisting poses, and inversions is very powerful for the health of the body and mind. Inversions are said to reverse the effects of gravity on the body, particularly on the internal organs. Inversions also increase blood flow to the brain, rejuvenating the brain, calming the mind, and awakening a sense of well-being.

The two most powerful poses in yoga, shoulder stand and headstand, are believed to benefit the health of the entire body and reverse the aging process. With the legs inverted in the air, the shoulder stand tones the thyroid glands in the neck. The thyroids are responsible for keeping hormonal levels balanced in the body. When hormones become imbalanced, the body deteriorates. This is why the shoulder stand is said to help reverse the aging process, as well as alleviate headaches, insomnia, depression, high blood pressure, and colds and illness. The headstand affects the pituitary and pineal glands in the brain and increases the oxygen content of the red blood cells. Yogic teachings say that if you practice headstands regularly, it will widen the horizons of your spirit. This means what once seemed impossible begins to seem possible. The reality is anything *is* possible.

The twisting poses in yoga are incredibly powerful for the internal organs. They are said to help wring out old blood and fluids from the liver, kidney, and spleen. As the organs are flushed of old blood, new oxygen-rich blood, brought in from the deep breathing during yoga practice, is able to flow into the internal organs, keeping them rejuvenated and toned. All of the poses, as well as the deep diaphragmatic breathing in yoga, also improve metabolism, aiding in weight loss and helping to maintain healthy weight.

It's also said that aging, as well as conditions like arthritis, occur when there is a lack of mobility and a depletion of the water element (*ojas*) in the body. Water is responsible for the transportation of every single cell in the body through the bloodstream, as well as the fluids of all the joints, muscles, and bones. Movement supports the flow of all of these fluids. This is why it's so important to eat water-rich foods like fruits and vegetables to keep your body as healthy and youthful as possible.

Mental Benefits

All of the yoga poses also have mental benefits as well. The connection to breathing is very powerful. Breathing is the thread of all of life and connects us to everyone and everything. When breathing is short, erratic, and choppy, our mind is scattered, distracted, and unfocused. But, when breathing is slow, deep, and rhythmic it calms the nervous system and awakens peacefulness, calmness, and evenness of mind, which, is one of the greatest benefits of yoga.

The reality is unless you are practicing a mind-body-breath practice like yoga, most people don't take the time to practice breathing. This is why going through the poses for 15 minutes to one hour is so beneficial—it gives you time to connect to your breath. This allows your mind to become calm, focused, and centered as your body feels healthy and well from the poses. We can only fully realize the benefits of anything when we make it a consistent practice in life, whether it is yoga, exercise, nutrition, meditation, prayer, playing an instrument, writing, or any other healthy living practice.

If you haven't started your yoga practice yet, now is the time. I was a little nervous about going to my first yoga class in 2001, but I went with a friend and I have been practicing yoga regularly ever since. I realized right away how amazing it was for me physically, mentally, emotionally, and spiritually. I had been exercising at a gym for years but had never felt as incredible as I did after my first yoga class. It was like everything in my body felt balanced, toned, cleansed, and renewed. Going to group classes with a teacher you enjoy is incredibly beneficial because you feel the positive energy of everyone around you practicing and doing their best. You also get to meet new people and develop wonderful friendships with those who are inspired to grow on the path of well-being, too.

There's no reason to be uncomfortable about going to a group class because yoga classes are all about creating a supportive, loving, nonjudgmental environment. But if you aren't comfortable attending a class yet, or there isn't one in your area, you can practice yoga at home. There are so many wonderful DVDs and downloadable online yoga classes, including my True Yoga classes, which are available at www.trueyogainc.com. To realize yoga's optimal benefits, a healthy practice consists of three to five sessions per week, but any time you practice yoga, you'll feel better.

Meditation and Healing the Mind

Meditation is one of the most powerful and positive practices for your life, and the mind is one of the most powerful instruments there is. Through quieting your mind and becoming aware of your thoughts you can begin to let go of unhealthy thinking and harness your mind and self for good. Many people think meditation is not thinking, but it is actually becoming aware of your thoughts so you can heal and let them go. The simple truth is we are either using the mind in a constructive way that supports our growth in a positive direction, or we are allowing mental chatter, worries, and concerns to be unhealthy or destructive. As your body becomes free of tension, your breath smooth and steady, and your mind still, you will be able to enter into the state of meditation with increasingly greater ease.

Yoga and meditation practice help to heal the subconscious mind by letting go of negative thoughts about yourself or others and awakening a healthy mind with loving and positive thoughts toward yourself as well as those around you. It is said that negative thoughts and thinking are the greatest obstacles on the spiritual path of well-being. Do you know there was a time, as infants and toddlers, that we had no negative or judgmental thoughts about anyone or anything? It is possible to reawaken those peaceful, loving thoughts. This doesn't mean you won't ever have a thought that feels egotistical or negative, but through the practice of yoga and meditation you can become instantaneously aware when you are having one of those thoughts about yourself or your neighbor and let it go. Private meditation and group meditation have helped me to heal through difficult experiences in my life, including the loss of my father. There was a time, after my father passed away, that I felt like I was dying almost every day because I felt so much pain from that loss in my life. In fact, during my first birthday after my father died I couldn't even eat because I was in so much physical and emotional pain. But the peacefulness that came from meditation, turning everything over to God, and feeling the love and support of positive people in my life allowed me to find eventual peace. It has been incredibly strengthening and has brought healing to my body, mind, and spirit. Even while writing this book and going through the Fresh Fruit Cleanse, I realized in a deeper way the healing power of yoga in all the ways it nourishes me through family, friends, meditation, and food.

How to Meditate

Meditation is often not easy at first, but as you continue to practice it will become easier. This is another reason why the practice of yoga poses is so beneficial: yoga helps to free the body of tension and calm the mind, preparing you to be able to sit still in meditation for an extended period of time.

It is best to meditate every day in the morning and the evening, but ultimately, any time is a good time to meditate. An ideal meditation practice may take anywhere from 15 to 30 minutes twice a day, increasing that time when you are able. It's also very powerful to meditate in a group. As a nun from the Self-Realization Fellowship once said to me, even meditating for five minutes each day is better than nothing.

The greatest teachings of meditation I've found have come from the teachings of Paramahansa Yogananda, one of the most incredible spiritual teachers of meditation in the 20th century. These at-home meditation lessons are available from the Self-Realization Fellowship (www.yogananda-srf.org). At their website, you can also find out if there is an SRF meditation group in your area.

The School of Metaphysics (www.som.org) is also an excellent resource for learning meditation. They offer many helpful books, CDs, DVDs, and online meditation classes. Visit their website to learn more about the School of Metaphysics and find out if there is one in your area. If possible, it is good to have a meditation teacher, someone who has been meditating for longer and can offer support and guidance along the way.

Healing Mantras

One of my favorite mantras to meditate on is the simple *I am*. *I am* is one of the most powerful mantras there is. The inhale is the breath of affirmation. This means as you breathe in, you affirm to yourself what you are, and as you exhale, you let go of any thoughts that don't support your highest self. When you are going through a yoga practice of sitting in meditation, you can inhale *I am*, and exhale out any thoughts that are not positive or loving about yourself or anyone else. As you inhale, think about what you are affirming to yourself. Perhaps you have been thinking something negative, like that you aren't beautiful or intelligent. These are the disempowering thoughts that are often in the subconscious mind, and they affect how we feel. Instead of affirming what you *don't* want to be, affirm what you *do* want to be or become.

Be still, and know that I am God.
—*Psalm 46:10*

Here are a few examples:

- Inhale: I am / Exhale: beautiful.
- Inhale: I am / Exhale: joyous.
- Inhale: I am / Exhale: peaceful.
- Inhale: I am / Exhale: awakening to the light of intelligence.
- Inhale: I am / Exhale: awakening to radiant health, well-being, and balance.
- Inhale: I am / Exhale: a healthy and beautiful expression of the light within my soul.
- Inhale: I am / Exhale: healthy and my body is beautiful.
- Inhale: I am / Exhale: igniting positive changes in my life and my life is growing in a positive way.

This mantra of *I am* will help you much in the same way purifying your body through the Fresh Fruit Cleanse will. It's so important to eat consciously and be aware of the thoughts you are having as you eat food. If you are continuously thinking something is going to make you overweight, then that is what will show up on your body. Everything is energy, and our mind affects our physical reality. No matter what you eat or drink, think positive thoughts to yourself about it, even if it's something you believe is unhealthy.

Here are some positive thoughts to have both during and after the Fresh Fruit Cleanse:

- This food is nourishing every cell of my body and awakening optimal health throughout my being.
- Each molecule of energy my body receives from this food will be spiritualized and metabolized in the best way possible for optimal health and well-being.

- Every morsel of food awakens beautiful energy and creates glowing beauty in every cell of my being.
- My body is in perfect balance and harmony, and each inhale and exhale brings optimal balance into my physical being and awakens radiant health.

The Fresh Fruit Cleanse and the recipes and nutrition in this book are the most healing nutritional program I have found for my own life. Eating like this is a way of life for me. That doesn't mean I don't have occasional indulgences, but I now have a health and wellness program that I can follow that helps me feel the best I can. There is always more to learn about enhancing health and well-being, but this is a good start. And for that I am eternally grateful.

17

Inspirations and Affirmations to Live By

Kindness is the light that dissolves all walls between souls, families, and nations.

—*Paramahansa Yogananda, spiritual guide and teacher, 1893–1952*

Be afraid of nothing. Hating none, giving love to all, feeling the love of God, seeing His presence in everyone, and having but one desire—for His constant presence in the temple of your consciousness—that is the way to live in this world.

—*Paramahansa Yogananda*

Be not conformed to this world: but be ye transformed by the renewing of your mind, that ye may prove what is that good, and acceptable, and perfect, will of God.

—*Romans 12:2*

Live each moment completely and the future will take care of itself. Fully enjoy the wonder and beauty of each moment.

—*Paramahansa Yogananda*

Be as simple as you can be; you will be astonished to see how uncomplicated and happy your life can become.

—*Parmahansa Yogananda*

Develop an attitude of gratitude, and give thanks for everything that happens to you, knowing that every step forward is a step toward achieving something bigger and better than your current situation.

—*Brian Tracy, self-help author, b. 1944*

Yes, there is Nirvanah: it is in leading your sheep to a green pasture, and in putting your child to sleep, and in writing the last line of your poem.

—*Kahlil Gibran, Lebanese American artist, poet, and writer, 1883–1931*

Not being beautiful was the true blessing...Not being beautiful forced me to develop my inner resources. The pretty girl has a handicap to overcome.

—*Golda Meir, fourth prime minister of Israel, 1898–1978*

The best things are nearest: breath in your nostrils, light in your eyes, flowers at your feet, duties at your hand, the path of God just before you. Then do not grasp at the stars, but do life's plain common work as it comes, certain that daily duties and daily bread are the sweetest things of life.

—*Robert Louis Stevenson, Scottish novelist, poet, and essayist, 1850–1894*

It's better to light a candle than to curse the darkness.

—*Chinese Proverb*

I slept and dreamt that life was joy. I awoke and saw that life was service. I acted and behold, service was joy.

—*Rabindranath Tagore, Bengali poet, novelist, musician, playwright, 1861–1941*

Our deepest fear is not that we are inadequate. Our deepest fear is that we are powerful beyond measure. It is our light, not our darkness, that frightens us most. We ask ourselves, "Who am I to be brilliant, gorgeous, talented, and famous?" Actually, who are you not to be? You are a child of God. Your playing small does not serve the world. There is nothing enlightened about shrinking so that people won't feel insecure around you. We were born to make manifest the glory of God that is within us. It's not just in some of us; it's in all of us. And when we let our own light shine, we unconsciously give other people permission to do the same. As we are liberated from our own fear, our presence automatically liberates others.

– Marianne Williamson, spiritual activist, writer, lecturer, and founder of the Peace Alliance, b. 1952

Finding Your Life's Purpose

So, how do you find your purpose in life? Finding your purpose is one of the most important quests you can have in this lifetime. When you find your purpose, you will be inspired to be healthy and well and to make the world a better place. The best advice I can give you, even if you have found your purpose in life, is to pray that you will continue to discover and be strengthened in that purpose according to your highest good and God's will. When you pray you are asking, seeking, and knocking, and the answer will be given to you. It may not always come all at once, but it will come.

You are today where your thoughts have brought you; you will be tomorrow where your thoughts take you.

—James Allen, British pioneer of the self-help movement, 1864–1912

Whether you are following the path of your passion in life, or not, there are going to be challenges. The important part is to realize you are surrounded by God's love and people in life who want you to succeed and be the best you can be. While there are challenges in life, there is always a way to get back up again and keep going and moving forward in the best way possible.

> Dream lofty dreams, and as you dream, so you shall become. Your vision is the promise of what you shall one day be; your ideal is the prophecy of what you shall at last unveil.
>
> —*James Allen*

There is a quote that has guided my life over the last ten years. It comes from the spiritual text, the Bhagavad-Gita, which is rich with spiritual wisdom and insight. It says, *"let the work alone be the joy, ne'er the fruits thereof."*

So, if you don't know what your purpose in life is yet, no worries. Keep praying and asking the questions and you will find what makes your soul and heart sing. Our work evolves over time. When you come from the place of love in life with all your work, you will be blessed and life will give to you. I believe we are here on this earth to serve and to live the purpose God intends for us. When you are living your divine purpose, your heart and soul will be filled with joy.

18

Conclusion

After a few days of the Fresh Fruit Cleanse, you will realize the impact food has on every aspect of your life, including how you look and feel. This is why, for optimal health, it's essential to follow a nutritious diet as well as exercise regularly and detoxify your body with an ongoing commitment to make healthier choices in life. Health is a journey. When you consider that you may have continued some unhealthy behaviors for years, it's understandable that letting go of these old patterns and healing may take time. Detoxification, which happens through the Fresh Fruit Cleanse and by continuing to live and eat in a healthy way, cleanses the bodies of impurities that have accumulated in the organs since birth.

As you continue to eat well, by following the recipes in this book and incorporating nutritious new recipes, and as you make a commitment to exercise regularly, perhaps practice yoga and meditate, and surround yourself with like-minded and positive people, you will find everything in your life will continue to improve and grow healthier. You needn't walk the path of wellness alone. There are loving, healthy people all around who are committed and inspired to walk the same spiritual path of well-being.

Does that mean you'll always make perfect choices? No. There will be times when you let yourself zag in life, and thank goodness for that. Life is meant to be lived and enjoyed, but it's important to realize that real and lasting joy doesn't—and never will—come from things like food, alcohol, cigarettes, or shopping.

Within the ten generations before your birth, over 1,000 people made their way through the world in order for you to be created. They are your parents, your grandparents, your great-grandparents, and on and on. Those souls walked the earth and their DNA flows in your veins, and they have a vested interest in your well-being and the evolutionary realization of your life at its fullest potential. Remember, there are now thousands of people, both living and transcended, who are cheering you on each step of the way.

So, with healthy living practices like the Fresh Fruit Cleanse, you can and will awaken to your true potential. Practice and all will come. This is life and it's time for all of us to break free of the bonds of fear, scarcity, and disbelief, and live to the fullest in the best way possible. This is the time to dream lofty dreams. And to know that as you dream so shall you become. This is the time to believe in God and in yourself and to know that anything you think in your heart you can become. Blessings and namaste.

Appendix

Testimonials

Meryl Blau *Miami, Florida*

I suffered from terrible constipation for about a year and a half. I eat a healthy diet and include plenty of fiber, so this was really frustrating. It began with all the changes in my body post-pregnancy. I did not want to live on medication in order for my body to function. A friend introduced me to the fruit cleanse as an alternative, and I was willing to try anything, especially if it meant avoiding more medication.

My husband and I did the cleanse together the week before Thanksgiving. It was an amazing experience. We felt completely revitalized and refreshed. I lost a few pounds but didn't notice any immediate change in my constipation issues, but as the next week went on I did, and I still do months later. It's the only thing that has worked.

My husband and I plan to do the 1-day cleanse every month or so this year, just because we know what a great effect it has on the body. Thank you, Leanne. You saved me from a lot of pain—and unnecessary medication!

Anietie *Dallas, Texas*

After the overly indulgent holidays, the Fresh Fruit Cleanse was the perfect way to reset my palate for healthy, nourishing foods in the new year. During the 3-day cleanse, I lost more than 3½ pounds. But the benefits weren't just physical. While cleansing, I took a much more mindful approach to eating that stays with me even now. I was inspired to pursue a healthier diet from that time onward. Two plums up for the Fresh Fruit Cleanse! Thanks, Leanne.

Abbe Timmons *Dallas, Texas*

I had been wanting to do a cleanse for a long time, so I was thrilled when Leanne let me be a part of hers. This was my first time doing a fruit cleanse. I had full intentions of using the recipes but realized I was just not organized enough to include them, so I opted for eating pieces of fresh fruit. This was easier for me to stick to, and I could eat while working. I also drank the detox tea every morning (which I loved and am still drinking). I think three days is a perfect length for a first cleanse. It was amazing how clear my mind was! I noticed that I slept very well and woke up feeling awake and light. I did go to a yoga class while cleansing, but I made sure not to overexert myself, and I did fine. After the cleanse, I felt great. It really put me on track for continuing to eat well.

Since the cleanse I find myself wanting an apple or pear for lunch instead of the heavy sandwich or fast food I used to eat. I will definitely continue to do the cleanse, probably the three-day cleanse at every change of season. Thanks again, Leanne!

Stephanie LaFlamme *Dallas, Texas*

I started the Fresh Fruit Cleanse on a Monday morning with a plan to do it for three days. However, I ended up feeling so great and was not at all hungry or anxious to stop that I extended it by two days. As the book suggests, I mentally prepared myself by thinking and reading about cleansing. I loved both the Detox Smoothie and the Green Protein Smoothie. I also loved eating fresh fruit with flax oil dribbled on top for a snack or a meal. Each afternoon I marinated tomatoes in olive oil, vinegar, garlic, salt, and pepper, so by the evening they were delicious and hearty enough to fill me up along with just some avocado.

I have two young children and a husband, so I was still preparing meals and snacks for then, but, amazingly, not snacking on their food wasn't as hard as I thought it would be. I was committed, and it felt really good.

My yoga practice on the fifth day of the cleanse was wonderful. I was full of energy and not weighted down by any heavy food.

On top of how great I felt, what I found most rewarding was the realization that I could stick to a program like this. Everything was delicious, and I carried over that feeling of serenity as I returned to my regular diet. It was an amazing experience. Thank you, Fresh Fruit Cleanse!

Logynn B. Northrhip *Austin, Texas*

My first day of the cleanse was my worst, because I went from having coffee every day to stopping cold turkey. I had a headache and was very sleepy and grumpy. All of this changed by day two. I could feel the fog lifting, and by day three I was alert and clear headed. I loved all of the recipes that I tried. I lost only a few pounds, but I was feeling better and better. I was on the cleanse for five days, and I can honestly say that I prefer this way of eating for most of the week. It is easy and healthy.

My favorite recipes were Coconut Mango Soup, Cold Tomato and Cucumber Soup, and Fruit Day Spaghetti with Sauteed Eggplant. I did the Fresh Fruit Cleanse during winter, and it was the warmer cooked foods that helped me to stay on the plan for so long. In fact, I did it for three days the following week, as well. Once I went back on my regular meals, I found I was not as in love with coffee as I once was—I kept thinking about Green Protein Smoothies!

Kaitlin Chu *Dallas, Texas*

I had been looking for a detox program to follow. The Fresh Fruit Cleanse is incredibly inviting and makes anyone feel that they are capable of taking on such a challenge. I love the cleansing effect of the Detox Blast Smoothie, and the rich vitality I feel after drinking the Green Protein Smoothie—it's great before or after a workout. The amazing thing about the recipes is that once you purchase a few of the ingredients, you start adapting mentally, and you want to continue mixing different fruits and flavors! Turmeric powder and cayenne pepper are now staples in my household. I have already passed on these recipes to two other families who have incorporated them into their lifestyles, as well! Thanks, Leanne.

David Tietje *Dallas, Texas*

I started this cleanse very reluctantly. Reading through the recipes and information seemed overwhelming and I wasn't sure I could even begin, but I had made a commitment and so I jumped in. I had intended to cleanse for only three days, but it wasn't as difficult as I had imagined, so I made it all seven days! I did not manage to follow the diet perfectly. I had some tortilla chips with the Tomato Basil Soup and a few other slips, but overall I think I did a good job.

Sometimes when you make a change, you try it out a few days and then go right back to your previous ways. So far it's been almost two months, and I have kept to the changes. I'm eating more consciously than ever before, and for that I am grateful. I seldom get headaches anymore, and I'm completely off soft drinks, which I was almost addicted to.

Rocio Morales *Round Rock, Texas*

Leanne Hall has made the Fresh Fruit Cleanse tasty, doable, affordable, and easy to follow. I never felt deprived or hungry, and I enjoyed the easy and delicious recipes. It was nice to get away from my usual diet, and I gained some healthy tips for improving my diet. No doubt I'll go back to cleansing during the change of seasons or just to give my body a boost.

References

Books

Balch, Pyllis A., CNC. *The Prescription for Nutritional Healing: The A-to-Z Guide to Supplements.* New York: Avery, 2002.

Condron, Daniel R. *Superconscious Meditation: Kundalini & the Understanding of the Whole Mind.* Windyville, MO: School of Metaphysics Publishing, 1998.

Daniels, Jennifer, M.D., and Mitra Ray, Ph.D. *Do You Have the Guts to Be Beautiful?* Seattle: Shining Star Publishing, 2008.

Garrison, Robert Jr., M.A., R.Ph., and Elizabeth Somer, M.A., R.D. *The Nutrition Desk Reference.* New Canaan, CT: Keats Publishing, 1995.

Kadans, Joseph M., N.D., Ph.D. *Encyclopedia of Fruits, Vegetables, Nuts, and Seeds.* West Nyack, NY: Parker Publishing, 1973.

Mosby, Karen, ed. *Fruit Day Cookbook.* Windyville, MO: School of Metaphysics Publishing, 2005.

Waton, Ronald R., ed. *Vegetables, Fruits, and Herbs in Health Promotion.* Boca Raton, FL: CRC Press, 2001.

Willett, Walter C., M.D. *Eat, Drink, and Be Healthy: The Harvard Medical School Guide to Healthy Eating.* New York: Free Press, 2001.

Woloshyn, Tom. *The Complete Master Cleanse: A Step-by-Step Guide to Maximizing the Benefits of The Lemonade Diet.* Berkeley, CA: Ulysses Press, 2007.

Candida

Msoffe, Peter M., and Mbilu, Z. M. 2009. The efficacy of crude extract of *Aloe secundiflora* on *Candida albicans*. *African Journal of Traditional, Complementary and Alternative Medicines* 6(4), 592–595.

Tips, Jack, N.D., Ph.D. *Conquer Candida and Restore Your Immune System. Copyright 1987, 1989.* Austin, TX: Apple-A-Day Press, 1995.

Cayenne

Willard, T. 2004. Herb profile: Cayenne. *Alive: Canadian Journal of Health and Nutrition* (260), 114–115.

Chia Seeds

Kreiter, T. (2005). Seeds of Wellness: Return of a Supergrain. *Saturday Evening Post* 277(b), 40–107.

Chocolate

Wolfe, David, and Shazzie. *Naked Chocolate*. San Diego, CA: Maul Brothers Publishing, 2005.

Coconuts

http://www.hailmerry.com

Gabbay, Simone. 2010. Coconut water: Elixir from the tropics. *Alive: Canadian Journal of Health and Nutrition* (337), 135–136.

Daily Values

U.S. Food and Drug Administration Food Labeling Guide (www.fda.gov).

The Dirty Dozen

http://www.ewg.org/foodnews/summary

Flax

Wasserman, Carole Anne. 2008. Flax, the new miracle food. *Macrobiotics Today*, 48(4).

Garlic

Is Raw Really Better? EN Weighs In on the Raw vs Cooked Debate. (2005). *Environmental Nutrition* 28(7), 7.

Insulin

http://www.endocrineweb.com/conditions/diabetes/diabetes-what-insulin

Maca

http://www.superfoods.co.za/maca.htm

Mattes, C. 2010. Maca. *Alive: Canadian Journal of Health and Nutrition* (332), 44–45.

Rona, Zoltan P., M.D. 2008. The wonders of maca. *Alive: Canadian Journal of Health and Nutrition* (309), 104–105.

Milk Thistle

Willard, Terry. 2009. Milk thistle. *Alive: Canadian Journal of Health and Nutrition* (317), 64–65.

Parasite Cleanse

"Homemade Colon Cleanse" (http://www.homemadecoloncleanse.net/parasite-cleanse.html)

"Your Liver, Parasites, and the Healing Crisis" (http://altered-states.net/barry/update200/index.html)

Protein

http://www.happycow.net/vegetarian_protein.html

Skin

Cajic, Natalie. 2010. Beauty from within: Skin supplements that activate beauty from the inside out. *Alive: Canadian Journal of Health and Nutrition* (338), 63–65.

Spirulina

Butler, G. 2004. Green means go. *Alive: Canadian Journal of Health and Nutrition* (257), 86–87.

Duelli, Nicole. 2008. Spirulina & chlorella. *Alive: Canadian Journal of Health and Nutrition* (314), 82–83.

http://www.herbwisdom.com/herb-spirulina.html

http://www.superfoods.co.za/spirulina.htm

Robb-Nicholson, Celeste. 2006. By the way, doctor. *Harvard Women's Health Watch* 14(3), 8.

Shyam, R., Singh, S. N., Vats, P., et al. 2007. Wheat grass supplementation decreases oxidative stress in healthy subjects: A comparative study with spirulina. *Journal of Alternative and Complementary Medicine* 13(8), 789–792.

Sugar

http://www.askdrsears.com/html/4/t045000.asp

http://www.ehow.com/facts_5206706_foods-containing-sucrose.html

http://www.sixwise.com/newsletters/2009/april/29/glucose-fructose-sucrose-whats-the-difference.html

Turmeric

http://www.kimberlysnyder.net/blog

Pantazis, P., Varman, A., Simpson-Durand, C., et al. 2010. Curcumin and turmeric attenuate arsenic-induced angiogenesis in ovo. *Alternative Therapies in Health and Medicine* 16(2), 12–14.

Lynde, M. 2007. Terrific turmeric. *Alive: Canadian Journal of Health and Nutrition* (294), 70–71.

About the Author

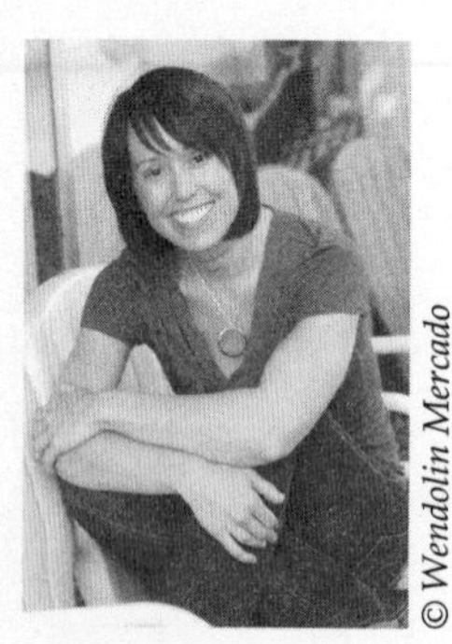
© Wendolin Mercado

LEANNE HALL has been following her passion for health, wellness, nutrition, yoga, meditation, and spirituality for over a decade. After graduating from Ohio University in 2000, she intended to develop a career in broadcast journalism, but found her true love for holistic health and wellness when she took her first yoga class in 2001. Since then, she has explored the world of nutrition, studying about many nutritional lifestyles, including cleansing, super foods, vegetarianism, veganism, and the raw foods diet. Her experiences have led her to her practice and passion for healthy food and nutrition. Leanne is the owner of True Yoga and the developer of *True Yoga Blog* (www.trueyogainc.com/blog) where she shares information and inspiration related to living a healthy and inspired life. She continues to be inspired to learn and study about the vast knowledge of nutritional well-being and its incredible power to promote healing physically, mentally, emotionally, and spiritually and looks forward to continuing to share her love for health and wellness with you on www.freshfruitcleanse.com and *True Yoga Blog*. Leanne can be reached via e-mail at leanne@trueyogainc.com.